Heart Disease

Pocket tutor

Heart Disease

Paul Morris MBChB MRCP BMedSci PhD
Specialist Registrar in Cardiology
Sheffield Teaching Hospitals NHS
Foundation Trust
Clinical Research Fellow
University of Sheffield
Sheffield, UK

David Warriner BSc MBChB MRCP DipSEM
Specialist Registrar in Cardiology
Sheffield Teaching Hospitals NHS
Foundation Trust
Sheffield, UK

Allison Morton BMedSci MBChB PhD FRCP
Consultant Cardiologist
Heartcare Western Australia
Bunbury, WA
Honorary Senior Lecturer
University of Sheffield, UK

Paul Mayhew BSc
Medical Writer
Berlin, Germany

JP
medical
publishers

© 2016 JP Medical Ltd.

Published by JP Medical Ltd, 83 Victoria Street, London, SW1H 0HW, UK

Tel: +44 (0)20 3170 8910   Fax: +44 (0)20 3008 6180

Email: info@jpmedpub.com   Web: www.jpmedpub.com

ISBN: 978-1-909836-32-7

British Library Cataloguing in Publication Data
A catalogue record for this book is available from the British Library

Library of Congress Cataloging in Publication Data
A catalog record for this book is available from the Library of Congress

Publisher:	Richard Furn
Development Editors:	Thomas Fletcher, Alison Whitehouse
Editorial Assistant:	Katie Pattullo
Design:	Designers Collective Ltd

Preface

Coronary heart disease is the commonest cause of death in the world. Many of the factors which place people at risk of coronary heart disease, such as physical inactivity, obesity, smoking and a diet high in fat and salt, are avoidable. A challenge for clinicians is that coronary heart disease develops silently over many years before manifesting as chest pain, heart attack, arrhythmia, heart failure or even sudden cardiac death.

Conditions such as hypertension, diabetes and hypercholesterolemia can be considered as silent killers because these also predispose to atherosclerosis, the underlying cause of coronary heart disease, and are associated with few, if any, symptoms.

Pocket Tutor Heart Disease reinforces important principles and improves understanding of the basic science and clinical management of coronary heart disease, from atherosclerosis to the complications of acute myocardial infarction. We hope that this deeper understanding enables all healthcare professionals to improve coronary heart disease prevention and care for their patients more effectively when the disease manifests clinically.

Lastly, a word on terminology: this book is called *Pocket Tutor Heart Disease* in the interests of brevity. The focus is upon coronary heart disease, its signs, symptoms, risk factors, presentations and complications. That is the scope of this book.

Paul Morris, David Warriner,
Allison Morton, Paul Mayhew
February 2016

Contents

Acknowledgements

Figures 1.28, 1.30, 1.31, 1.35, 1.39, 1.40 and 1.41 are reproduced from: Mann J, Marples D. Eureka Physiology. London: JP Medical, 2015.

Figures 1.42, 1.43, 1.44, 1.45, 1.46, 1.47, 1.48, 1.49, 1.50 and 1.51 are reproduced from: Davison A, Milan A, Phillips S, Ranganath L. Eureka Biochemistry & Metabolism. London: JP Medical, 2015.

Figure 2.2 is reproduced from: Craythorne E, Daly M-L. Pocket Tutor Dermatology. London: JP Medical, 2015.

Figure 2.12 is reproduced from: Parker S. Eureka General Surgery & Urology. London: JP Medical, 2015.

Figure 2.13 is copyright of Sam Scott-Hunter and reproduced from: Tunstall R, Shah N. Pocket Tutor Surface Anatomy. London: JP Medical, 2012.

Figure 2.14 is reproduced from: Borooah S, Wright M, Dhillon B. Pocket Tutor Ophthalmology. London: JP Medical, 2012.

Figure 2.19 is reproduced from: James S, Nelson K. Pocket Tutor ECG Interpretation. London: JP Medical, 2011.

First principles

The heart beats from the 3rd week of embryonic life until the moment of death – more than 3 billion times in a lifetime. Only the size of a fist and weighing 300 g, the heart pumps > 7000 L of blood per day through nearly 100,000 km of blood vessels.

The main purpose of the cardiovascular system (**Figure 1.1**) is to transport substances around the body, including:

- Oxygen (O_2) and nutrients (e.g. glucose, amino acids) to tissues
- Waste products [e.g. carbon dioxide (CO_2), urea and lactate] from tissues
- Fluids and electrolytes
- Hormones to target organs
- White blood cells
- Clotting factors and platelets
- Heat, to aid thermoregulation.

1.1 Cardiovascular anatomy

HEART

The heart is composed of muscle arranged around a framework of fibrous tissue and is the size of a fist. The two atria collect blood and fill the two ventricles, which pump blood into the pulmonary and systemic circulations (**Figure 1.2**). Its four valves prevent blood flow in the wrong direction.

Cardiomyocytes are the main cells of the heart (see page 28). The interstitium between them contains collagen, elastin, fibrous connective tissue, blood and lymphatic vessels.

Surface anatomy and relations

The heart is in the middle mediastinum with its apex pointing inferolaterally (**Figures 1.3** and **1.4**). It is posterior to the sternum, costal cartilages and left lung pleura and superior to the left diaphragm. Structures adjacent to the posterior heart

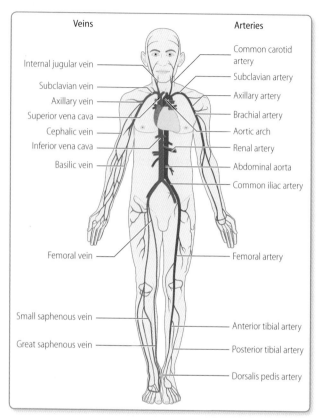

Figure 1.1 The cardiovascular system.

are the thoracic vertebrae, esophagus and descending aorta (**Table 1.1**).

Chambers and valves

The heart has four muscular chambers, each connected to a great vessel. The four valves lie between the ventricles and atria and the ventricles and the great arteries (**Figure 1.5**).

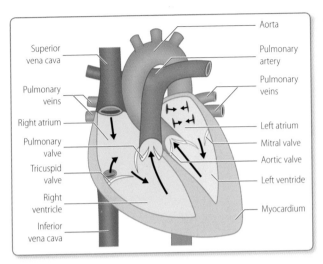

Figure 1.2 The heart.

Left atrium

The mitral orifice and valve separate the left atrium and ventricle. The atrium receives its blood supply from the left circumflex coronary artery. The left atrial appendage or left auricle is a muscular out-pouching continuous with the left atrium. The left and right atria are separated by the interatrial septum.

Mitral valve

The mitral valve prevents blood regurgitating back into the left atrium during systole. It has two leaflets (i.e. it is bicuspid):

- The anterior leaflet attaches to the anterior aspect of the mitral orifice
- The posterior leaflet attaches to the posterior orifice

The free edges of the leaflets are attached to the chordae tendinae, which attach to the left ventricular papillary

> ### Clinical insight
>
> Ventricular dilatation or ischemic damage to the papillary muscles can disrupt the subvalvular apparatus, allowing regurgitation to occur

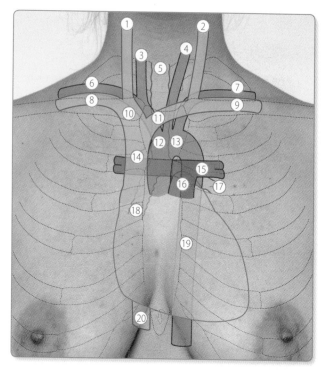

Figure 1.3 Surface anatomy of the heart and great vessels. ①, right internal jugular vein; ②, left internal jugular vein; ③, right common carotid artery; ④, left common carotid artery; ⑤, trachea; ⑥, right subclavian artery; ⑦, left subclavian artery; ⑧, right subclavian vein; ⑨, left subclavian vein; ⑩, right brachiocephalic vein; ⑪, left brachiocephalic vein; ⑫, brachiocephalic trunk; ⑬, arch of aorta; ⑭, superior vena cava; ⑮, left pulmonary artery; ⑯, pulmonary trunk; ⑰, left main bronchus; ⑱, right main bronchus; ⑲, descending aorta; ⑳, inferior vena cava.

Guiding principle

The force countering systemic circulation (i.e. resistance) is five times higher than that of the pulmonary circulation. Consequently, the walls of the left ventricle are three times thicker (6–12 mm) than the right ventricle

muscles. This subvalvular apparatus prevents valve prolapse during systole.

Left ventricle

The left ventricle is an elongated inverted cone that

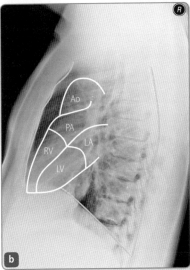

Figure 1.4 Radiographs showing the borders of the heart and great vessels. (a) Frontal view. The right heart border (red) is formed mainly by the right atrium. The left heart border is formed mainly by the left ventricle (LV, green) and the left atrium (LA, blue). The inferior surface (against the diaphragm) represents the right ventricle (RV). The vena cava (pink) is above and below the right heart border, and the aortic arch (yellow) and pulmonary trunk (purple) are above the left atrium. (b) Lateral view. The anterior, posterior and inferior relations of the heart (orange) are formed by the sternum or left lung pleura, thoracic spine and diaphragm, respectively. Ao, aorta; PA, pulmonary artery.

is circular in cross-section (**Figure 1.6**). Its internal surface is heavily trabeculated by muscle fibers (**Figure 1.7**).

The mitral valve chordae tendinae attach to an anterior and posterior papillary muscle.

Cardiac surface	Main structure	Extracardiac relation
Anterior (sternocostal)	Right ventricle	Sternum
		Costal cartilages
		Left lung pleura
Posterior (base)	Left atrium	Thoracic vertebrae
		Esophagus
		Descending aorta
Inferior	Left ventricle	Left hemidiaphragm
Apex	Left ventricle	Sternum
		Costal cartilages
		Left lung pleura

Table 1.1 The structures and borders of the four cardiac surfaces.

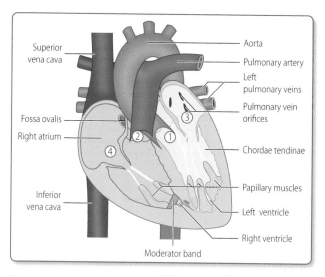

Figure 1.5 Anatomy of the heart valves. ① Aortic valve. ② Pulmonary valve.
③ Mitral valve. ④ Tricuspid valve.

Figure 1.6 Transthoracic echocardiogram showing the circular left ventricle (LV). The lower pressure right ventricle (RV) accommodates the higher pressure left ventricle.

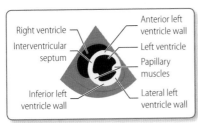

Right ventricle

Interventricular septum

Inferior left ventricle wall

Anterior left ventricle wall

Left ventricle

Papillary muscles

Lateral left ventricle wall

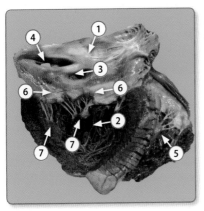

Figure 1.7 An exploded view of the left atrium (LA) ① , left ventricle (LV) ② and mitral valve ③ . The left atrial appendage ④ orifice and a pulmonary vein ⑤ are visible in the LA. Trabeculations of the LV are coarser than those of the right ventricle ⑥ . The mitral valve leaflets ③ are tethered to the papillary muscles ⑦ by the chordae tendinae. Courtesy of Dr K Suvarna.

Blood enters the left ventricle through the mitral valve and exits via the aortic valve. The outflow tract is posterior to the right outflow tract, which 'wraps' around the aorta. Blood supply is from the left anterior descending (LAD) artery and its diagonal branches.

Aortic valve and aortic root

The aortic valve has three semilunar cusps (**Figure 1.8**). The aortic root is directly above the valve, and has three dilations, or sinuses, two of which are the origin of coronary arteries.

The ascending aorta continues superiorly and toward the right before bending leftwards and posteriorly, arching over the left lung hilum.

Figure 1.8. A transthoracic echocardiogram showing the aortic valve in cross-section.

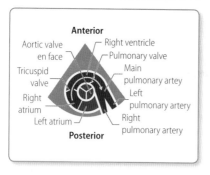

Right atrium

The right atrium receives deoxygenated blood from the superior and inferior venae cavae and coronary venous blood through the coronary sinus. The smooth posterior surface is separated from the trabeculated anterior surface by the crescent-shaped crista terminalis muscle.

The trabeculated right atrial appendage – the auricle – projects from the superoanterior segment of the atrium.

Tricuspid valve

The tricuspid valve has anterior, posterior and septal leaflets. Their free edges are attached to the ventricular walls by the chordae tendinae and papillary muscles, which are smaller than the left subvalvular apparatus.

Right ventricle

The right ventricle, like the left, is an elongated inverted cone shape, but operates at a much lower pressure. As a result, the left ventricle and interventricular septum bulge into the right ventricular cavity (**Figure 1.6**).

The moderator band is a ridge of muscle that extends from the septum to the anterior wall at the base of the papillary muscle. It is part of the electrical conduction pathway that ensures the right-sided papillary muscles contract before the ventricle does, to ensure the tricuspid valve is braced for systole.

Pulmonary valve

The pulmonary valve is a tricuspid, semilunar valve at the apex of the right ventricular outflow tract.

Blood supply and drainage

Coronary heart disease (CHD) is a disease of the coronary arteries, and clinical understanding requires a thorough knowledge of the heart's blood supply.

Arterial supply

The left coronary artery (LCA) usually originates from the left coronary sinus, and the right coronary artery (RCA) emanates from the right coronary sinus.

Clinical insight

Myocardium has a relative lack of collateral arterial connections; arterial occlusion quickly results in ischemia and infarction.

Clinical insight

CHD kills more people worldwide than any other disease. It occurs when an atherosclerotic plaque disrupts and occludes the coronary arterial lumen (see page 228).

The arteries run along the epicardial surface of the heart until they branch into smaller arteries, which penetrate and supply the myocardium. They are effectively end arteries, with only minimal anastomoses between them.

Left coronary artery

The LCA passes behind the pulmonary artery and along the atrioventricular groove, where it divides into the left anterior descending and circumflex arteries (**Figure 1.9**).

Figure 1.9 The left coronary artery.
(a) Relations with other cardiac structures.
(b) Left-sided angiogram of the left coronary artery. A coronary catheter is sitting in the aortic root, where it injects X-ray contrast material into the left main stem.
①, coronary catheter; ②, diagonal artery; ③, left anterior descending artery; ④, obtuse marginal artery; ⑤, circumflex artery.

The LAD artery roughly follows the line of the anterior septum down to the apex. It provides diagonal branches to the left ventricle laterally, and septal branches inferiorly to the interventricular septum.

The circumflex artery winds around the left lateral surface of the heart in the atrioventricular groove toward the inferior surface. Distally, it anastomoses with right-sided vessels on the inferior surface of the heart. Along its length, it supplies obtuse marginal branches that supply the high lateral wall of the left ventricle.

Right coronary artery

The RCA usually supplies the sinoatrial (SA) node, right ventricle, atrioventricular node and inferior surface of the left ventricle (**Figure 1.10**). It travels in the right atrioventricular groove to the inferior surface of the heart. From here, it usually supplies the

Figure 1.10 The right coronary artery. (a) Relations with other cardiac structures . (b) Angiogram taken from in front of the patient. The right coronary artery ① winds around the right atrioventricular groove, from which it branches to the sinoatrial (SA) node ② and right ventricle ③ before travelling down the inferior surface of the heart. A catheter ④ is visible in the descending aorta and in the aortic root at the right coronary ostium.

posterior descending artery lying along the line of the inferior interventricular septum. Proximally, the RCA supplies a branch to the SA node. It also provides a branch to the right ventricle in its midsection.

Arterial dominance

Arterial dominance is determined by the artery that supplies the AV node (and usually the posterior descending artery):

- 75% are right-dominant (RCA)
- 15% are left-dominant (LCA)
- 10% are codominant.

Venous return

The great cardiac vein drains the anterior, posterior and lateral myocardial walls. It runs alongside the LAD artery and then in the left atrioventricular groove and empties into the right atrium through the coronary sinus. The middle cardiac vein begins at the apex, accompanies the posterior descending artery and drains into the coronary sinus.

Many right ventricular veins drain through the small cardiac vein directly into the right atrium.

The cardiac conduction pathway

The cardiac conduction pathway governs the route of myocardial depolarization and therefore pattern of its contraction (**Figure 1.11**). It is formed by:

- The SA node – spontaneously depolarizing pacemaker cells (see page 34) in the superior posterior right atrium
- Atrial cardiomyocytes that propagate depolarization
- The atrioventricular node – normally the only electrical connection between the atria and the ventricles
- The bundle of His and Purkinje fibers – specialized conduction fibers in the ventricular septum and ventricles, respectively
- Ventricular cardiomyocyte propagation

Other than at the AV node, insulating fibrous tissue prevents conduction between the atria and ventricles. The node

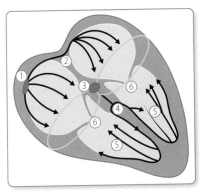

Figure 1.11 The conduction pathways of the heart. The sinoatrial (SA) node ①, Bachmann's bundle ②, atrioventricular node ③, bundle of His ④, which divides into left and right bundle branches. Purkinje fibers ⑤ rapidly conduct to the ventricles. Fibroannular rings ⑥ (shown in yellow) insulate the ventricles from the atria.

causes a pause in conduction, ensuring that ventricular filling is complete before contraction begins.

The bundle of His

The bundle of His descends in the ventricular septum and branches toward the right and left ventricles. The left bundle further divides into an anterior and a posterior branch, which subsequently form Purkinje fibers. These innervate the myocardium so that ventricular contraction starts at the apex and spreads to the base. This allows the efficient ejection of blood and ensures that the papillary muscles contract in time to prevent tricuspid or mitral valve regurgitation.

The pericardium

The pericardium is a double-membrane sac covering the heart and proximal segments of the great vessels. The outer tough fibrous pericardium protects the heart. The serous pericardium has two layers with a cavity in between:

- Parietal pericardium – a layer of mesothelial cells continuous with the fibrous pericardium
- The pericardial cavity containing a lubricating fluid to reduce friction
- Visceral pericardium that lines the epicardium.

It also contains lymphatic tissue with a role in immune function.

The phrenic nerve innervates the fibrous and parietal layers, whereas the visceral layer is innervated by the autonomic nervous system (ANS).

VESSELS

Ventricular contraction forces blood through the arteries under high pressure. As arteries branch, the number of blood vessels increases but their individual calibre decreases. Vast networks of capillaries perfuse tissues, in which substances are exchanged between blood and cells. Veins return blood to the heart under low pressure.

All vessels are cylindrical tubes of connective tissue and endothelial cells, and large vessels also have muscular, nervous, lymphoid and even vascular tissue.

Structure

All blood vessels, except capillaries, have three layers (**Figure 1.12**).

Tunica intima

This innermost layer is a single layer of endothelial cells, supported by a thin layer of connective tissue – lamina propria – and longitudinal elastic fibers, the internal elastic lamina. The luminal surface of the endothelial cells is in contact with blood in the lumen.

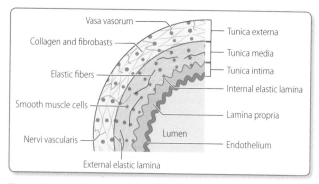

Figure 1.12 General structure of the walls of blood vessels. Vaso vasorum are the blood vessels to blood vessels; nervi vascularis are the nerves innervating vessels.

Tunica media

The middle layer consists of smooth muscle cells and elastic fibers in a circumferential arrangement. The smooth muscle is innervated by the sympathetic nervous system to control tone, i.e. vessel diameter. The external elastic lamina provides additional support

Tunica externa

This outermost layer is mainly collagenous connective tissue and is fused with surrounding connective tissue to anchor vessels in place.

Types

The structure of each vessel type reflects its function (**Table 1.2**).

Elastic arteries

These are the major proximal arteries: the aorta and the brachiocephalic, carotid, subclavian, iliac and pulmonary arteries. Their tunica media contain many elastic fibers, which convert the intermittent, pulsatile blood flow from heart contraction into the continuous flow allowing constant tissue perfusion. They absorb energy during systole and discharge it in diastole.

Muscular arteries

Muscular – or distributing arteries – distribute blood to the resistance arterioles. They have multiple layers of smooth muscle in their tunica media, and include the radial, mesenteric and femoral arteries.

Arterioles

Arterioles are known as resistance vessels because they regulate systemic vascular resistance (**Figure 1.13**). They

> ### Clinical insight
> Arteries become less elastic and more resistant as they age, causing an increase in systemic blood pressure from around 110 mmHg (average) at the age of 20 years to around 150 mmHg at 80 years.

contain one or two layers of smooth muscle that are autoregulating and affected by neuroendocrine control (see page 49).

Arteriolar muscular tone is the primary controller of perfusion as these vessels supply capillary beds.

Vessel(s)	Main function	Description
Aorta and other elastic arteries	Compliance: distensibility and elasticity convert pulsatile to continuous flow	Thick media layer, rich in elastic fibers, collagen and smooth muscle
Muscular artery	Distribution of blood to the arterioles	Thick media layer, rich in smooth muscle
Arteriole	Generate peripheral resistance and control blood flow	Layers of smooth muscle
		Richly innervated by the autonomic nervous system
Capillary	Exchange of gases, nutrients and waste products	Single layer of endothelial cells
Venule	Collection of capillary blood	Thin, poorly developed tunica media
Vein	Acts as capacitance vessel (blood reservoir)	Thin media layer, with scant elastic and smooth muscle fibers
		Compliant and contains valves
Vena cava	Returns blood to the right atrium	Very large vein in which flow is influenced by action of respiratory and cardiac pumps

Table 1.2 Structure and function of major vessels.

Capillaries

Capillaries consist of a single endothelial cell layer. They are 5–20 µm in diameter and about 1 mm long. However, they have a very large combined cross-sectional area, which results in a slow transit time. Known as exchange vessels, they are the site of gas, nutrient and waste product exchange between blood and tissues.

The microcirculation

The microcirculation is the functional unit of small vessels perfusing an organ or tissue (**Figure 1.14**). It consists of the:

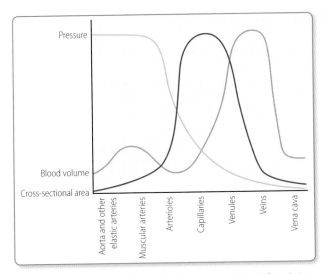

Figure 1.13 Pressure, blood volume and surface area at each level of circulation. The largest pressure drop occurs at the resistance vessels (arterioles), capillaries have the largest surface area and veins (capacitance vessels) hold the most volume.

Figure 1.14 The microcirculation. ①, The simple branched microcirculation architecture present in most tissues. ②, Central metarteriole, a thoroughfare channel with branching capillaries. ③, Direct atrioventricular anastomosis found in cutaneous tissues.

- Terminal arterioles
- Capillary bed
- Post-capillary venules
- Metarterioles, which bypass the capillary bed.

Microcirculation is regulated by terminal arteriolar tone, extrinsically by sympathetic innervation, and intrinsically, via autoregulation.

Precapillary sphincters   These rings of vascular smooth muscle encircle the entrance to capillary beds. They control whether blood enters that bed or is shunted via metarterioles to post-capillary venules.

Venules and veins

Post-capillary venules join to form larger venules, which join to form veins.

Venules and veins have a much thinner tunica media and less smooth muscle than arteries and arterioles. They are thin, compliant and lack elastic recoil. Consequently, they accommodate large increases in blood volume with minimal increase in pressure. The large combined cross-sectional area means resistance is low, so their low pressures are sufficient to return blood to the heart.

The large capacity of veins acts as a reservoir of blood and is regulated by the ANS. Sympathetic activation, for example, results in venous constriction, increasing venous return (and central venous pressure). Venous return is aided by the skeletal-muscle pump, where skeletal muscular contraction forces blood toward the heart and venous valves prevent backflow.

Key regional vascular anatomy

Carotid arteries

The right common carotid artery is a branch of the brachiocephalic artery. The left emerges directly from the aortic arch. The common carotid arteries bifurcate at the level of the C3–C4 vertebrae into the internal and external carotid arteries (**Figure 1.15**).

The internal carotid artery   The internal carotid artery enters the skull through the carotid canal, passes through the cavernous

Figure 1.15 Arteries of the neck and face. (1), superficial temporal artery; (2), maxillary artery; (3), masseter muscle; (4), facial artery; (5), internal carotid artery; (6), occipital artery; (7), lingual artery; (8), carotid bifurcation; (9), superior thyroid artery; (10), thyroid cartilage (vertebral level C5); (11), scalenus anterior; (12), transverse cervical artery; (13), suprascapular artery; (14), vertebral artery; (15), common carotid artery; (16), thyrocervical trunk; (17), subclavian artery; (20), internal thoracic artery. The best position to palpate the carotid artery is lateral to the larynx at the level of the thyroid cartilage ⊗.

sinus and supplies the ophthalmic artery. Its terminal branches are the middle and anterior cerebral arteries.

The external carotid artery   The external carotid artery supplies parts of the thyroid, larynx, tongue and superficial neck, face and head (**Table 1.3**).

Carotid sinus   The carotid sinus is a dilation in the carotid artery, just below the bifurcation of the common carotid artery. It contains baro- and chemoreceptors involved in the regulation of blood pressure and ventilation (see page 59).

Branch	Supplies:
Superior thyroid artery	Larynx Thyroid gland
Ascending pharyngeal artery	Skull base
Lingual artery	Tongue Mouth floor
Facial artery	Superficial face
Occipital artery	Back of the head Sternomastoid muscles
Posterior auricular artery	Scalp and ear
Maxillary artery (terminal branch)	Meninges, maxilla and mandible
Superficial temporal artery (terminal branch)	Scalp

Table 1.3 The main braches of the external carotid artery, inferior to superior.

Clinical insight

The carotid sinus is prone to atherosclerosis due to non-laminar blood flow. Atheroma can thromboembolize to cause a stroke. Risk is assessed via ultrasound.

The gut

The arterial supply to the gut is from branches of the abdominal aorta (**Table 1.4**), which enters the abdomen behind the diaphragm at the level of the T12 vertebra. It then descends, to the left of the midline, and divides at L4 into the common iliac arteries.

Clinical insight

Thromboembolic disease of arteries supplying the gut can lead to bowel ischemia and infarction which requires emergency surgery.

Renal vessels The renal arteries arise as lateral branches from the aorta at the level of the L1 vertebra (**Figure 1.16**). They are large in caliber – 0.5–1 cm – reflecting the high level of kidney perfusion, about a quarter of total cardiac output. They divide into segmental, lobar, interlobar and arcuate arteries before becoming the afferent arterioles supplying the glomeruli.

Branches	Supplies
Segmental arteries	Vertebrae
Celiac and mesenteric arteries	Gastrointestinal tract
Renal arteries	Kidneys
Adrenal arteries	Adrenal glands
Gonadal arteries	Gonads

Table 1.4 Branches of the abdominal aorta

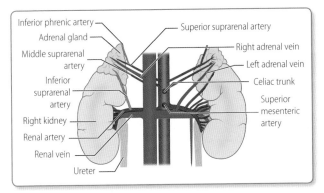

Figure 1.16 The arteries and veins of the kidneys and adrenal glands. The major vessels are the inferior vena cava and the abdominal aorta.

The renal veins mirror the arteries along their course.

Adrenal vessels The adrenal glands also have a rich blood supply via their superior, middle and inferior supra-renal arteries. These usually arise from the inferior phrenic artery, aorta and renal arteries, respectively. The right adrenal vein drains into the inferior vena cava, whereas the left drains into the left renal vein.

Clinical insight

Atherosclerosis or congenital diseases such as fibromuscular dysplasia can narrow the renal arteries. Such stenosis is a cause of resistant hypertension, kidney failure and atrophy.

1.2 Development of the cardiovascular system

The heart and vessels form by vasculogenesis, *de novo* vessel formation from endothelial precursors called angioblasts in the embryo. This stem cell budding is guided by genetic signals that orientate the direction and extent of growth. Further growth of small vessels occurs via angiogenesis, where vascular cells arise from already formed endothelial cells.

Development of the heart

The heart is the first organ to function and starts beating 3 weeks after fertilization. It initially forms a single tube that then folds, loops and is divided by septae to form the four chambers and major vessels.

> **Guiding principle**
>
> In embryology:
> - Superior = cranial
> - Inferior = caudal
> - Anterior = ventral
> - Posterior = dorsal

Endocardial tubes

The three layers of cardiac tissue – endocardium, myocardium and epicardium – develop from cardiogenic mesoderm at the cranial end of the embryo:

- **Day 18**: bilateral clusters of angioblasts form paired endocardial (heart) tubes
- **Embryonic folding** aligns these tubes in the midline on the ventral surface
- **Day 21**: the two tubes fuse to form a single-chambered heart with five segments that develop into chambers (**Figure 1.17** and **Table 1.5**). Myocyte rhythmic activity begins before tube fusion
- **By week 4** contraction starts pumping blood in a caudal to cranial direction.

Looping

On **days 23–28**, the growing tube folds and loops to the right (**Figure 1.17b**) to produce:

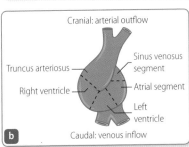

Figure 1.17 The heart tube. (a) Day 21: the heart tube has five distinct segments and four transitional zones. (b) Day 23–28: the tube folds and loops to resemble the mature heart.

Segment	Eventual structure
Truncus arteriosus	Aortic and pulmonary outflow tracts
Bulbis cordis	Right ventricle
Ventricular	Left and right ventricles
Atrial	Left and right atria
Sinus venosus	Coronary sinus and right atrium

Table 1.5 Structures originating from the five segments of the primitive heart tube.

- Caudal segments: sinus venosus and primitive atria
- **Cranial segments:** primitive ventricle and truncus arteriosus (the outflow tracts).

Once aligned, the atrial and ventricular segments begin to expand, differentiate and trabeculate. Externally, the heart starts to resemble the mature structure but internally remains a relatively simple folded, looped tube until the chambers and outflow tracts are divided by septation, the formation of tissue septa.

> ## Guiding principle
>
> The precision of heart tube looping is critical for the correct formation of chambers, vessels, and valves.

Atrioventricular septation

From **day 26**, cells surrounding the atrioventricular canal start to infiltrate the cardiac jelly, the gelatinous substance in-between the myocardium and endocardium. These form endocardial cushions – tissue that grows horizontally to form the valves and vertically, the septa.

Ventricular septation

Ventricular septation begins on **day 25**. From the apex of the cardiac loop, between the left ventricle and the bulbus cordis (the primary heart loop), the muscular interventricular septum starts to develop toward the endocardial cushions. The trunco-conal septum extends inferiorly into the ventricular cavity to form the membranous portion of the interventricular septum.

Ventricular septation is completed in **week 7** when the primary muscular septum, the truncoconal septum and the atrioventricular endocardial cushions fuse. This joins the ventricular and outflow tract septae, which connect the left and right ventricles to the aortic and pulmonary outflow tracts, respectively.

Atrial septation

Atrial septation starts around **day 30**, when the septum primum descends from the roof of the atrium toward the endocardial cushions. In the fetus, blood shunts through the orifice primum. Once this is obliterated by the fusion of the septum primum and the endocardial cushions, the second ostium develops.

The septum secundum then develops directly to the right of the septum primum. Both septae have posteroinferior windows that together form the foramen ovale. This flap valve allows right-to-left blood flow (**Figure 1.18**) and closes when systemic blood pressure increases after birth.

Dorsally, the left horn of the sinus venosus forms the coronary sinus, which empties into the right atrium. The right horn becomes incorporated into the structure of the right atrium.

The primordial pulmonary vein merges with the left atrium in week 5. By **week 8**, all four pulmonary veins are absorbed.

Outflow tract septation

The truncus arteriosus is a common outflow tract. From week 5, along its length endocardial ridges form in a spiral arrangement. When these meet in the middle and fuse, they form a septum that separates the aortic outflow tract from the pulmonary outflow tract). The same process is responsible for development of the aortic and pulmonary semilunar valves, and is completed by the end of **week 8**.

> **Clinical insight**
>
> Failure of septation results in septal defects between the cardiac chambers, a common congenital heart disease

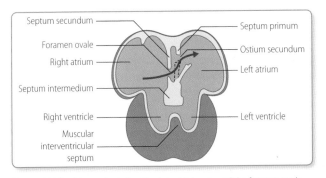

Figure 1.18 Fetal heart circulation. The interatrial septa and the foramen ovale flap valve (black dashed line). The rigid septum secundum grows alongside the septum primum. Fast flowing blood from the ductus venosus is directed across the atrial septae through the foramen ovale flap valve (red arrow). The valve closes after birth due to increased left atrial pressure.

The conduction tissue

Conduction tissue cells develop from the transitional zones of the heart tube. Regular contraction begins on **day 22**, before conduction tissues are formed. By the **7th week**, cells in the primitive atrium start to differentiate into the specialized pacemaker cells of the SA node, and cells of the sinus venosus into the AV node.

Development of vessels

Most vessels form by budding vasculogenesis from angioblasts. This initially forms a network of capillaries, with larger vessels formed as key pathways are enlarged. Further capillaries form via angiogenesis.

Arterial development

Arteries develop from the six, more ventral, paired aortic arches, along with the metabolic needs of the developing fetus (**Figure 1.19**):

- The first three arches develop into the arteries of the head and neck
- The 4th pair develop into the aortic arch and subclavian artery
- The 5th arches completely regress
- The 6th right arch develops into the right pulmonary artery, and the left arch develops into the left pulmonary artery and the ductus arteriosus.

> ### Clinical insight
>
> In the future, improved understanding of coronary artery embryology may allow the use of regenerated tissue to bypass sections blocked (i.e stenosed) by atherosclerosis. Current materials used in coronary artery bypass grafts or stenting are prone to restenosis.

Coronary arteries

The coronary arteries originate from ventricular endocardial cells, at the right and left aortic sinuses of Valsalva.

Venous development

Veins mainly form from three bilateral veins in **weeks 4–8**:

- The cardinal system drains the head and body
- The umbilical system supplies O_2– and nutrient-rich blood from the placenta

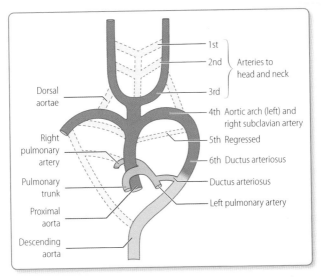

Figure 1.19 The aortic arches and dorsal aortae. The six arches develop and (some) regress at different times. Pair 1 regress but remnants form the adult maxillary and stapedial arteries. The 3rd pair form the carotid arteries. Pair 4 form the arch of the aorta (left) and the right subclavian artery. The 5th pair regress. Pair 6 contribute to the pulmonary arteries with the left also forming the ductus arteriosus. The dorsal aorta fuse in the midline forming the descending aorta.

- The vitelline system initially drains the yolk sac but develops into the hepatic, portal and superior mesenteric veins.

1.3 Cardiovascular physiology

Key physiological and biochemical processes to understand in CHD are:
- Electrophysiology
- The autonomic control of the heart
- The cardiac cycle
- Blood flow
- Blood pressure
- Hemostasis
- Lipid and cholesterol metabolism.

Vascular inflammation and immunology, particularly endothelial cell involvement, are also central in the development of
atheroma, but are beyond the scope of this book.

Electrophysiology

The cardiac cycle starts with the spontaneous initiation of an
action potential – the cardiac impulse – by pacemaker cells of
the SA node. This wave of depolarization then conducts along
specialized conduction tissues and cardiomyocytes, causing
them to contract.

Cardiomyocytes

Cardiomyocytes are branched, tubular cells with a central
nucleus (**Figure 1.20**). They connect end to end at intercalated
discs. The discs contain desmosomes that anchor cells together,
and gap junctions, which allow action potentials to conduct
freely between cells.

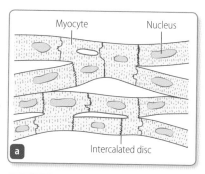

Figure 1.20 Cardiac
muscle. (a) Cardiomyocytes
are branched, nucleated,
elongated, tubular cells
joined at intercalated
discs. (b) Close up of
an intercalated disc.
Desmosomes anchor cells,
and gap junctions allow
ions to pass freely between
cells.

Resting membrane potential

Myocardial membranes have an electric charge – a resting potential of –90 mV, which allows them to conduct the cardiac impulse. This reflects unbalanced ion concentrations and selective membrane permeability maintained by membrane ion channels.

The main ions involved are the cations K^+, Na^+ and Ca^{2+} (**Table 1.6**):

Stage 1

Membrane-bound ion pumps actively pump K^+, Na^+ and Ca^{2+} out of the cell to make a small contribution to the RMP (**Figure 1.21**):

- Na^+/K^+-ATPase pumps three Na^+ ions out of the cell and two K^+ ions into the cell
- Ca^{2+}-ATPase pumps Ca^{2+} out of the cell and into the sarcoplasmic reticulum
- The Na^+–Ca^{2+} exchanger exchanges three Na^+ ions for one Ca^{2+} ion.

Stage 2

The membrane is permeable to K^+ but not other ions. K^+ therefore passively diffuses out of the cell, down its concentration gradient, increasing the intracellular negative charge.

Stage 3

K^+ efflux continues until equilibrium is reached between

> ### Guiding principle
>
> A myocyte with a resting membrane potential is polarized, i.e. there is a significant electrochemical gradient across the cell membrane. Depolarization triggers myocardial contraction.

Cation	Intracellular concentration (mmol/L)	Extracellular concentration (mmol/L)
K^+	150	4
Ca^{2+}	10^{-4}	2
Na^+	15	145

Table 1.6 Intracellular and extracellular concentrations of important cations.

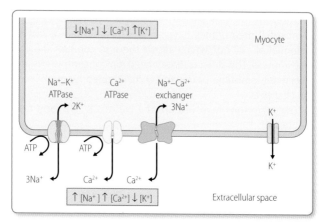

Figure 1.21 The resting membrane potential across the cardiomyocyte membrane. The three ion pumps (left) consume ATP to generate steep ionic concentration gradients. The membrane is permeable to K^+ but less permeable to other ions. Therefore, K^+ diffuses passively down its concentration gradient (right), leaving less positive charge (i.e. a net negative charge) on the inside of the cardiomyocyte.

its concentration gradient and its electrochemical gradient. This equilibrium potential (E) is determined by ionic charge and the concentration gradient. For K^+, E_K is around −96 mV.

Stage 4

The membrane potential (E_m) is equal to the sum of the equilibrium potentials of all the ions, proportional to their ability to cross the membrane (conductance, g):

$$E_m = (g_K \times E_K) + (g_{Ca} \times E_{Ca}) + (g_{Na} \times E_{Na})$$

This is predominately determined by E_K, as K^+ has the highest conductance. Hence overall RMP is close to E_K.

Gated ion channels

The cycles of depolarization and repolarization are controlled by membrane ion channels (**Table 1.7**). Ion channels are 'gated'

Channel	Current	Function
Fast Na+ channel	I_{Na}	Rapid influx of Na+
Slow Na+ channel	I_b	Slow influx of Na+
'Funny' Na+ channel	I_f	Generates AP in pacemaker cells
Slow L-type Ca2+ channel	I_{Ca-L}	Prolongs AP in non-pacemaker cells
		Initiates AP in pacemaker cells
Transient T-type Ca2+ channel	I_{Ca-T}	Helps initiate AP
Inwardly rectifying K+ channel	I_{ir}	Maintains resting membrane potential
Transient outward K+ channel	I_{to}	Contributes to phase1 of AP
Delayed rectifier K+ channel	I_{Kr}	Contributes to repolarization

Table 1.7 Types of cardiomyocyte ion channel; AP, action potential.

Gating mechanism	Stimulus	Example
Voltage-gated channels	Electrical potential	Generation of action potentials
Ligand-gated channels	Ligand binding	Hormones and neurotransmitters
Receptor-coupled channels	Physical stimulus	Myocardial stretch

Table 1.8 Different gating mechanisms of ion channels.

in that they are activated (open) or inactivated (closed) by local factors such as voltage, ligand binding or receptor activation (Table 1.8).

Movement of charged particles, ions, generates an electrical current. Most of the current of depolarization is from Na+ influx (i.e. I_{Na}), which occurs until Na+ channels are deactivated.

Cardiomyocyte depolarization

The cardiomyocyte action potential has five phases (0–4) controlled by ion channel activation and inactivation (**Figure 1.22**). Phase 4 corresponds to diastole and phases 1 and 2 to systole.

Phase 4: resting

The membrane is permeable to K+ and relatively impermeable to other ions. Cardiomyocytes are held at RMP, polarized between –90 and –95 mV.

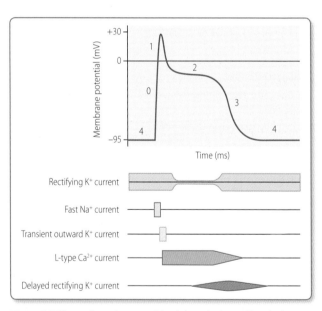

Figure 1.22 The cardiac action potential and the activation and inactivation of gated ion channels. The phases are 0, depolarization; 1, transient partial repolarization; 2, plateau; 3, repolarization; and 4, resting.

Phase 4 ends when a depolarizing electrical stimulus is conducted to the myocyte from a neighbouring cell. If it increases the membrane potential to –60 mV, an action potential (phase 0) is triggered.

Phase 0: depolarization

The threshold potential activates voltage-gated fast Na^+ channels and Na^+ ions rush into the cell, down a steep concentration gradient. I_{Na} rapidly increases the membrane potential to around +30 mV, when fast Na^+ channels abruptly inactivate.

Phase 1: transient partial repolarization

Voltage-gated, transient outward K^+ channels activate to allow a brief efflux of K^+ (I_{to}). This causes a brief partial repolarization.

Phase 2: plateau

Voltage-gated L-type Ca^{2+} channels activate and inactivate slowly, which prolongs inward Ca^{2+} current (I_{Ca}); this sustains the action potential for around 250 ms and triggers myocyte contraction.

Toward the end of phase 2, Na^+–Ca^{2+} exchangers allow slow entry of Na^+, extending the plateau phase.

Ca^{2+} and Na^+ influx is opposed by outward rectifying K^+ currents.

Phase 3: repolarization

As the L-type Ca^{2+} channels inactivate, delayed rectifying K^+ channels open. The now unopposed K^+ efflux causes rapid repolarization.

> ### Clinical insight
>
> Calcium channel blockers (e.g. verapamil and diltiazem) block L-type Ca^{2+} channels to shorten phase 2. They are negative ionotropes, i.e. they reduce cardiac contractility.

Refractory periods

The absolute refractory period is the time during phases 1 and 2 in which another action potential cannot be initiated. It is due to inactivation of fast Na^+ channels, which are not reactivated until phase 3. The relative refractory period is the time during their reactivation, when depolarization can occur but depends on the magnitude of the stimulus and the number of reactivated channels (**Figure 1.23**).

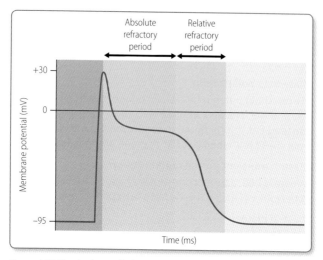

Figure 1.23 The absolute and relative refractory periods of an action potential in a cardiomyocyte.

Clinical insight

Drugs that block K⁺ channels (e.g. amiodarone) prolong phase 3 and the refractory period. They are useful in alleviating the symptoms of certain re-entry tachycardias.

Pacemaker depolarization

Pacemaker cells are cardiomyocytes that can spontaneously depolarize, found in the SA and AV nodes and conducting tissues. This *automaticity* – regular, spontaneous firing – is due to:

- A less negative resting potential ($E_m = -60$ mV)
- Leaky Na⁺ channels.

A relatively high Na⁺ permeability means they slowly depolarise until a threshold at –20 mV. This opens voltage-gated Ca²⁺ and slow Na⁺ channels, causing cation influx and an action potential spike (**Figure 1.24**).

Pacemaker potentials

The rate of inward Na⁺ and Ca²⁺ currents (I_{Na} and I_{Ca}) during phase 4 determines the rate of action potential generation and therefore heart rate.

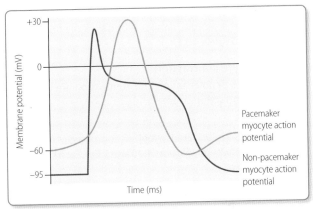

Figure 1.24 The action potentials of a pacemaker and a non-pacemaker cardiomyocyte. In a pacemaker cell, the resting potential (phase 4) is less negative and constantly drifts toward the firing threshold.

Pacemaker hierarchy

Multiple pacemaker sites provide a 'back up', though the fastest pacemaker functioning – the SA node in health – always assumes overall control. The more distal the pacemaker (relative to the SAN), the slower its intrinsic rate (**Table 1.9**).

Conduction pathway

The atrioventricular fibrous skeleton prevents the wave of depolarization spreading into the ventricles. The AV node is normally the only electrical connection from the atria to the ventricles. The node slows conduction, allowing complete

Pacemaker site	Intrinsic rate (depolarizations/min)
Sinoatrial node	100
Atrioventricular node	40–60
Bundle of His	30–40
Ventricles	≤ 30

Table 1.9 The hierarchy of pacemakers and their intrinsic heart rates.

atrial emptying into the ventricles. Depolarization then spreads rapidly down the septum via specialized Purkinje fibers in the bundle of His (**Figure 1.11**).

Cardiomyocyte contraction

Cardiomyocyte depolarization and contraction are linked via excitation–contraction coupling.

Myofibrils

Myocytes contain elongated myofibrils composed of functional units called sarcomeres (**Figures 1.25** and **1.26**). Each sarcomere

Figure 1.25 The sarcomere. (a) The sarcomere is bound by the Z lines – formed by the arbed ends of thin actin filaments. The filaments project centrally, where they interdigitate with thick myosin filaments. This gives the striated appearance of cardiomyocytes, defined by the M line, the H zone and the A and I bands. (b) Actin–myosin interaction.

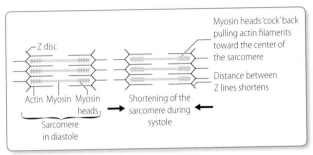

Figure 1.26 Sarcomeres and the sliding filament mechanism of myocardial contraction. Within the sarcomere, the central thick myosin filaments are surrounded by the thin actin filaments. Contraction of the many myocardial sarcomeres underlies contraction, and causes the H band to disappear, the A band to increase and the I band to shorten.

is bounded at each end by a Z line and contains contractile filaments made of the proteins actin and myosin. Peripherally, actin thin filaments attach to the Z line. Centrally, myosin thick filaments interdigitate (i.e. overlap) with the actin filaments.

Sarcolemma

The cell membrane – the sarcolemma – invaginates deeply into the myocyte around the Z lines to form T tubules. These are closely associated with sarcoplasmic reticulum, which contains intracellular stores of Ca^{2+}. This enables the rapid coupling of membrane (i.e. T tubule) depolarization with the release of Ca^{2+} from the sarcoplasmic reticulum to stimulate myofibril contraction.

Myofibril contraction

Thin filaments consist of actin, tropomyosin and troponin complexes (**Figure 1.27**).

- Troponin T attaches each troponin complex to the tropomyosin
- Troponin I inhibits the binding of myosin heads to actin
- Troponin C binds to Ca^{2+}.

The binding of Ca^{2+} to troponin C exposes the myosin-binding site, allowing actin–myosin cross-bridges to form.

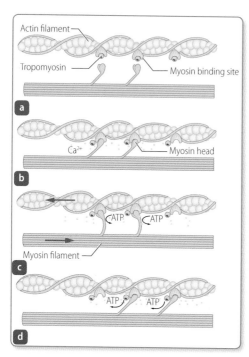

Figure 1.27 Mechanism of myocardial contraction. (a) Myosin-binding sites on actin filaments are blocked by tropomyosin. Ca²⁺ released after depolarization binds to troponin. (b) Troponin changes conformation, exposing the binding site. Myosin heads bind actin. (c) Power stroke occurs as myosin heads pull filaments and shorten the sarcomere. (d) Myosin heads reset and can rebind.

Labels in figure: Actin filament, Tropomyosin, Myosin binding site, Ca²⁺, Myosin head, ATP, ATP, Myosin filament, ATP, ATP

Clinical insight

The regulatory troponin complex is found in cardiac and skeletal muscle, but not (vascular) smooth muscle. Subunits T and I are only found in cardiomyocytes whereas C is also found in skeletal muscle. Troponin T and I blood levels are indicators of myocyte damage associated with myocardial infarction.

The sliding filament model of contraction The myosin 'power stroke' pulls the filaments so that they slide in opposite directions; this sliding shortens the sarcomere and in turn contracts the myocardium. Cycles of myosin-head binding to actin, contracting, disconnecting and then reattaching – a 'ratcheting' effect – progressively shorten the sarcomere as long as intracellular Ca²⁺ remains high. Both contraction and relaxation are energy dependent

(ATP consuming). In the heart this is a continual cycle hence the large concentration of mitochondria and glycogen stores.

Inotropism

Inotropism is the ability of an agent to affect muscle contractility (see page 46); positive inotropes enhance contractility and negative inotropes reduce contractility.

Autonomic control of the heart

The cardiovascular center is a collection of nuclei in the medulla oblongata, and is the branch of the ANS responsible for cardiovascular homeostasis and control. It receives sensory input from peripheral chemo- and baroreceptors, and higher control from the thalamus, hypothalamus and cerebral cortex (**Figure 1.28**). Through its modulated output it regulates:

- Heart rate (see page 47)
- Cardiomyocyte contractility (see page 46)
- Global blood flow (see page 49)
- Blood pressure (see page 58).

The sympathetic nervous system

Sympathetic signals are transmitted from pre-ganglionic neurons in the lateral thoracic and lumbar spinal cord (levels T1–L2). These synapse with post-ganglionic neurons within the right and left paravertebral ganglia (the sympathetic chains).

Sympathetic nerves innervate the atrial and ventricular myocardium, SA node, AV node and conduction tissues. They release noradrenaline (norepinephrine), which – along with adrenaline (epinephrine) in the bloodstream – activates β_1 adrenoreceptors in the heart.

Effects

Activation increases intracellular cyclic AMP (cAMP) and protein kinase A activation, causing changes in ion channel gating (**Table 1.10**), and thereby increases:

- Heart rate, i.e. chronotropicity
- Contractility, i.e. inotropicity
- Myocardial relaxation, i.e. lusitropicity
- Conduction through the AV node, i.e. dromotropicity.

Inputs:
- Sensory chemoreceptors and baroreceptors of the carotid and aortic bodies and proprioceptors of muscle
- Higher centers: cerebral cortex, hypothalamus and limbic system

Vagus nerve

Cardiovascular center of medulla

Preganglionic sympathetic nerves

Blood vessel

Outputs:
① Sympathetic nerves to SA and AV node: ↑impulses, ↑heart rate
② Sympathetic nerves to cardiomyocytes: ↑impulses, ↑contractility and stroke volume
③ Vagus nerve to SA and AV node: ↑impulses, ↓heart rate
④ Sympathetic nerves to vascular muscle: ↑impulses, ↑tone

Figure 1.28 The cardiovascular center of the medulla is responsible for the global control of heart rate, contractility and stroke volume, as well as vascular tone, the core determinant of blood pressure.

The parasympathetic nervous system

Efferent parasympathetic innervation of the heart is through the right and left vagus nerves (cranial nerve X), which originate in the nucleus ambiguous of the medulla oblongata. Pre- and post-ganglionic neurons synapse very close to the heart. Post-ganglionic neurons primarily innervate the atrial myocardium, SA node and AV node.

Channel	Change	Effect
Na^+ and Ca^{2+} channels	Activates	Increases phase 4 pacemaker currents and therefore heart rate
L-type Ca^{2+} channels,	Augments	Increases Ca^{2+} influx and therefore contractility (i.e. positive inotropicity)
Ca^{2+} pumps	Augments	More rapid Ca^{2+} clearance, which accelerates myocardial relaxation
Delayed rectifying K^+ channels	Augments	Shortens action potential duration

Table 1.10 Noradrenaline (norepinephrine) induced changes in membrane ion transport.

Vagal activation releases acetylcholine, which binds to muscarinic M_2 receptors, antagonizing cAMP production and protein kinase A activation. Vagal activation also results in K^+ channel activation and hyperpolarization of the myocyte membrane.

The parasympathetic nervous system reduces heart rate by reducing pacemaker potentials.

Clinical insight

Atropine blocks muscarinic acetylcholine receptors to reduce parasympathetic activation.

Guiding principle

At rest, parasympathetic (i.e. vagal) tone dominates the control of heart rate. During activity, vagal tone is reduced, and during exercise, sympathetic activity dominates.

The cardiac cycle

The cardiac cycle is the series of the events occurring every heat beat (**Figure 1.29**, **Table 1.11**).

Atrial systole

Atrial contraction (systole) is the active phase of ventricular filling that follows passive filling. At rest, it contributes 10–20% of total end-diastolic volume. This contribution decreases as the heart rate increases.

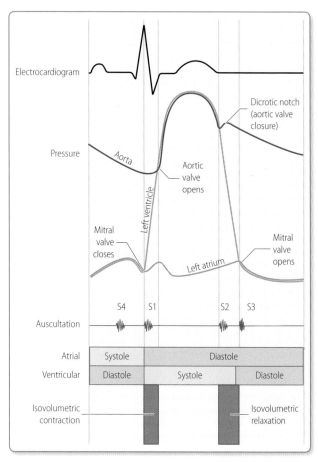

Figure 1.29 The cardiac cycle can be interpreted by electrocardiography, blood pressure dynamics and heart sounds.

A small pressure wave – the *a* wave – is detectable in the veins during this phase, as the atria are continuous with the great veins which do not have valves.

Atrial systole indirectly contributes to cardiac output as ventricular stroke volume is proportional to end-diastolic volume.

Heart sound	Mechanism	Timing	Circumstance
1st (S1)	Atrioventricular valve closure	Immediately before the carotid pulse	Normal
2nd (S2)	Semilunar valve closure	Immediately after the carotid pulse	Normal
3rd (S3)	Rapid early (passive) ventricular filling	Shortly after S2	Can be normal in young fit people but is also a sign of increased end-diastolic pressure, which occurs in heart failure
4th (S4)	Atrial systole against stiffened ventricle	Shortly before S1	Indicates stiffened (hypertrophied) ventricular walls

Table 1.11 The physiological basis of the heart sounds.

Ventricular systole

During ventricular systole:
- Ventricles contract
- Atrioventricular valves close (heart sound S1)
- Semilunar valves open
- Blood is ejected.

As the atrioventricular valves bulge into the atria, they produce a c pressure wave in the venous pulse when they close.

Ventricular pressure increases

The semilunar valves remain closed until the ventricular pressure exceeds the aortic and pulmonary artery pressures. This phase is called isovolumetric contraction because the ventricular pressure increases without any change in ventricular volume.

Ventricular ejection

Once the semilunar valves open, the pressure gradient across the valves is minimal and blood is powerfully ejected into the aorta and pulmonary arteries.

Atrial diastolic fillixng occurs during ventricular systole with a corresponding increase in atrial pressure (the *v* wave).

Ventricular diastole

During ventricular diastole:

- Ventricles relax
- Semilunar valves close
- AV valves open.

Ventricular systole continues until arterial pressures are slightly greater than ventricular. This allows a very brief reversal of flow that closes the semilunar valves (S2).

Ventricular relaxation

Ventricular pressure continues to decrease after the semilunar valves close. Ventricular volume is unchanged until the AV valves open, hence this phase is isovolumetric relaxation time. Ventricular relaxation is not passive, and active recoil of the ventricles helps to suck in blood during the next phase.

Atrioventricular valves open

The AV valves open as soon as atrial pressure exceeds ventricular, just after the point of peak atrial filling and pressure (the *v* pressure wave). Atrial pressure decreases rapidly. Ventricular filling is rapid at first and then slows as the pressure gradient declines.

Finally, atrial systole starts the next cycle.

Blood flow

At rest, total blood flow – cardiac output (CO) – is about 5 L/min. This can increase to 30 L/min during strenuous exercise. Both the total and local flow of blood are closely regulated to match global and local metabolic need.

Global control – the cardiovascular center

The cardiovascular center controls the rate and force of heart contraction and global vascular tone (see **Figure 1.28**).

Cardiac output

CO = heart rate (HR) x stroke volume (SV)

Therefore, the cardiovascular center controls total blood flow by adjusting heart rate (see page 47) or stroke volume.

(see page 47)

Stroke volume

Stroke volume is the volume of blood ejected with each heartbeat:

SV = end-diastolic volume (EDV) – end-systolic volume (ESV)

It is influenced by preload, myocardial contractility and afterload.

The ejection fraction (EF) is the percentage of blood ejected from the ventricle with each heartbeat. It is normally 50–70% but is reduced in heart failure.

$$\text{Ejection fraction (\%)} = \frac{SV}{EDV} \times 100$$

Cardiac preload Preload is end-diastolic ventricular pressure. An increase in preload increases end-diastolic and stroke volume.

The myocardium is at its most stretched at the end of diastole, which has two effects:
- More active actin–myosin cross-bridges form
- The affinity between Ca^{2+} and troponin C increases.

This is the basis for the Frank–Starling law: 'the mechanical energy discharged during ventricular systole is a function of initial fiber length', i.e. more myocardial stretch leads to a more forceful contraction (**Figure 1.30**). This is how:
- Left and right circulations equalize
- Exercise increases venous return and therefore CO
- Reduced venous return (e.g. hemorrhage) decreases CO.

Venous muscular tone can also affect venous return:
- An increase – e.g. sympathetic activation – increases venous return
- A decrease in tone decreases venous return.

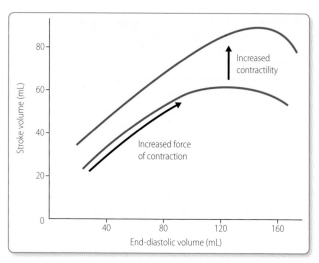

Figure 1.30 The Frank–Starling curve. An increase in end-diastolic volume results in a greater stroke volume. In the physiological range, the curve is steep as ventricles are particularly sensitive to changes in end-diastolic volume. Beyond the physiological range, the curve plateaus; further increases in end-diastolic volume do not increase stroke volume. The effect of raised contractility (often referred to as increased sympathetic tone) is demonstrated in the upper curve.

Contractility Contractility is the force of myocardial contraction, independent of preload. Inotropes affect contractility (**Table 1.12**) and are also the name of a class of drugs with positive inotropic effects ((e.g. digoxin; see page 156).

A positive inotropic agent – such as sympathetic activation or increased myocardial stretch – increases cardiomyocyte contraction, usually by increasing Ca^{2+} influx, which causes more actin–myosin cross-bridges to form.

Sympathetic activation increases contractility and heart rate via β_1 adrenoreceptors (see page 39). An increase in contractility shifts the Frank–Starling curve upwards.

Parasympathetic activation reduces rate but has no effect on contractility due to minimal parasympathetic innervation of myocardium.

Positive inotropes	Negative inotropes
Increase contractility	Decrease contractility
Sympathetic nervous activation Hormones, e.g. adrenaline (epinephrine) and thyroxine Serum ions (Ca^{2+}) β_1 agonists (e.g. dobutamine, isoprenaline and adrenaline) Phosphodiesterase inhibitors (e.g. milrinone)	General ill health (e.g. myocardial ischemia, acidosis and hypoxia) β_1 antagonists (beta-blockers) Calcium channel blockers

Table 1.12 Positive and negative inotropes.

Afterload Afterload is the ventricular tension required to eject blood against aortic or pulmonary artery pressures. An increase in afterload increases end-systolic volume and reduces stroke volume.

Tension is a factor of volume and pressure, and is therefore increased in conditions of ventricular dilatation. It is also increased by arterial hypertension and aortic stenosis.

Heart rate

As heart rate affects cardiac output and therefore blood pressure, the mechanisms controlling it and blood pressure are integrated. Sympathetic activation increases heart rate *and* contractility, as increasing the rate alone would decrease diastolic filling time and therefore end-diastolic volume (preload).

Guiding principle

An increase in central venous pressure increases cardiac output by:

- Frank–Starling's law – increased cardiomyocyte stretch causes increased contraction
- Bainbridge's reflex – right atrial stretch receptors increase sympathetic activation to the heart.

Peripheral signals to the cardiovascular center include pressure and chemical sensors in the carotid and aortic bodies:

- Baroreceptor activation (by being stretched) results in vagal activation and bradycardia
- Chemoreceptor stimulation, for example via low O_2 or glucose or raised CO_2, also leads to bradycardia, though the effect is less direct.

Hormones such as thyroxine and its metabolites increase heart rate. Extreme cold causes a reduction in heart rate, and higher body temperatures result in an increase in heart rate.

Total peripheral resistance

Total blood flow is also affected by total peripheral resistance (TPR), which is the sum force opposing blood flow, determined by the diameter of resistance vessels. This is dependent on vascular tone, the degree of smooth muscle contraction, and therefore constriction, of a vessel. Therefore global blood flow is also affected by changes in vascular tone. This is affected by innervations from the ANS and global hormones.

Vascular tone is also locally controlled by hormones and autoregulation – an intrinsic response of vascular muscle to maintain tone.

Vascular smooth muscle

Vascular smooth muscle contraction – like all muscle – involves Ca^{2+} release and the sliding filament model (see page 38). However, vascular contraction is slower and sustained compared to cardiac or skeletal muscle. It always has some degree of 'tone'. Unlike cardiac muscle, it lacks the troponin complex and cells are not arranged into a striated pattern.

Contraction occurs in response to electrical, mechanical or chemical stimulation:
- Membrane depolarization
- Stretch
- Receptor binding

Stimulation causes Ca^{2+} influx from the extracellular space and Ca^{2+} release from sarcoplasms:

1. Ca^{2+} binds to the protein calmodulin
2. Ca^{2+}-calmodulin complex activates myosin light chain kinase (MLCK)
3. MLCK phosphorylates myosin light chains
4. Actin–myosin crossbridges form and contraction occurs

Cycles of sliding filament contraction progressively shorten the myofibrils as long as intracellular Ca^{2+} remains high. Ca^{2+}ATPase and Na^+ Ca^{2+} exchanger membrane proteins actively remove Ca^{2+}.

Vascular tone

Vascular tone is proportional to the intracellular Ca^{2+} concentration. This is influenced globally by autonomic control and hormones and locally by chemicals and intrinsic autoregulation.

Extrinsic control of vascular tone This is affected by external factors:

- Vasoactive chemicals in the blood
- ANS activity (which releases vasoactive chemicals)
- Variations in membrane receptors for afferent nerves or hormones.

Vasoactive chemicals Vasoactive compounds work via four main mechanisms: three different G-protein linked signal transduction pathways (Gq, Gs and Gi), and nitric oxide (**Table 1.13**). Nitric oxide is one of the few gas signaling molecules.

Pathway	Examples	Mechanism	Effects
Gq-protein coupled	Catecholamines (adrenaline, noradrenaline–epinephrine, norepinephrine) angiotensin II, thromboxane A_2, endothelin I, vasopressin	Gq-protein linked receptor activates phospholipase C and diacylglycerol, causing Ca^{2+} release and myosin light chain phosphorylation	Vasoconstriction, membrane depolarization, Ca^{2+} sensitization
Adenylate cyclase (Gs- and Gi-coupled)	Catecholamines (via β_2 adrenoreceptors), adenosine, acetylcholine, prostacyclin	Gs-protein linked receptor activates adenylate cyclase to convert ATP into cAMP, which inhibits MLCK, reducing contractility	Vasodilation
	Catecholamines (via α_2 adrenoreceptors)	Gi-protein linked receptor inhibits adenylate cyclase, reducing cAMP, increasing MLCK activity	Vasoconstriction

Table 1.13 *Continued...*

Pathway	Examples	Mechanism	Effects
Nitric oxide	NO	Activates guanylate cyclase to convert GTP into cGMP, which inhibits Ca^{2+} influx, inositol triphosphate synthesis, membrane depolarization and increases myosin light chain dephosphorylation	Vasodilation
Sympathetic nerves: catecholamine release	α_1 receptor	Gq-protein linked receptor (see above)	Vasoconstriction
	α_2 receptor	Gi-protein linked (see above)	Vasoconstriction
	β_2 receptor	Gs-protein linked receptor (see above)	Vasodilation (primary action)
Parasympathetic nerves: acetylcholine release	Muscarinic M_3 receptors	Gq-protein linked receptor (see above)	Vasoconstriction (primary action, secondary effect)
	Muscarinic M_3 receptors	NO release (secondary action, principal effect) (see above)	Vasodilation (genitals, salivary glands and bladder)

Table 1.13 Mechanisms of vasoactive compounds. ATP, adenosine triphosphate. cAMP, cyclic adenosine monophosphate. GTP, guanosine triphosphate. cGMP, cyclic guanosine monophosphate. MLCK, myosin light chain kinase. NO, nitric oxide.

It is synthesized by endothelial cells – stimulated, for example by acetylcholine released by parasympathetic efferent neurons. It diffuses through vascular myocyte membranes to cause vasodilation.

ANS activity Generally, sympathetic adrenergic activation (via α receptors) vasoconstricts systemic vessels to increase TPR and therefore blood pressure, and cholinergic activation (via muscarinic receptors) stimulates sweating and dilates skin arteries. Most blood vessels have very little parasympathetic innervation. At rest, vagal tone dominates in the heart, whereas sympathetic tone dominates in vascular smooth muscle.

Intrinsic control of vascular tone Autoregulation is the intrinsic response of arteriolar smooth muscle to changes in perfusion or blood constituents in order to moderate local blood flow. Different networks can have different responses due to receptor variation. For example, hypoxia in the pulmonary circulation causes vasoconstriction, to match ventilation and perfusion; elsewhere it induces vasodilatation in an attempt to correct the abnormality.

The myogenic response Increased blood flow/pressure activates stretch receptors, causing reflex vasoconstriction and a decrease in local flow. This myogenic response maintains constant flow despite fluctuating mean arterial blood pressure (**Figure 1.31**).

Metabolic adaptation Increased cellular metabolism produces metabolites that are vasodilators, thereby matching blood flow to metabolic demand. They include K^+ ions, adenosine and CO_2.

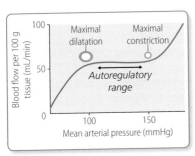

Figure 1.31 Myogenic autoregulation. Within the autoregulatory range a rise in pressure in the arterioles perfusing a tissue will cause reflex constriction, which increases resistance and maintains constant blood flow through the tissue.

Coronary blood flow

Myocardium has a high metabolic rate, reflected in its large numbers of mitochondria, and receives a high blood flow via an extensive capillary network. It is the most efficient organ at extracting O_2 from blood – about 70% that enters its circulation. Therefore, it relies on metabolic adaptation to match blood flow and O_2 supply. Its resting blood flow of 200–250 mL/min can increase to 1 L/min during exercise.

Contrary to other organs, coronary blood flow is impeded during systole and enhanced during diastole, particularly on the more muscular left side. The transmural pressure generated by systole compresses subendocardial arterioles so that myocardium is not perfused. Some systolic perfusion does occur in the outermost (i.e. subepicardial) myocardium, where transmural pressure is lower.

> ### Clinical insight
>
> The heart is unique in its efficiency in extracting O_2 from blood, which it does at a nearly constant maximum rate. Increasing blood flow is the only way to meet increased O_2 demand.

Left coronary artery flow

The highest LCA flow occurs during diastole (**Figure 1.32**). The lowest is during the isovolumetric phases of systole, when ventricular pressure is high but coronary flow is low.

Right coronary artery flow

Right ventricular myocardial perfusion is more consistent as wall tension is much lower than in the left.

Coronary flow reserve

This is the ratio of maximal to resting flow velocity. It is reduced in patients with significant, flow-limiting CHD and in those with microvascular disease.

Velocity is measured with an intracoronary Doppler wire during coronary angiography. Maximal velocity is induced pharmacologically, usually with adenosine. The ratio is calculated as the hyperemic flow velocity divided by baseline velocity.

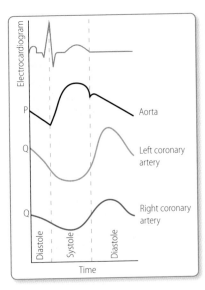

Figure 1.32 Coronary blood blow (schematic representation). Aortic pressure (P) peaks in systole; left coronary artery (LCA) flow (Q) peaks in diastole, due to high systolic resistance caused by compression of vessels in the ventricular wall. This effect is less in the right coronary artery (RCA) as right ventricular pressures are lower.

Hemodynamics

Hemodynamics is the study of physical laws governing blood flow.

Pressure, flow and resistance

The heart is an intermittent pump, generating pressure (P) to drive blood flow (Q) through the circulation against the force of resistance (R):

$$\Delta P = QR$$

This can be rearranged:

$$Q = \frac{\Delta P}{R}$$

i.e. an increase in driving pressure, or a reduction in resistance to flow both increase blood flow.

Applying this to the circulatory system:

- Flow (Q) is cardiac output (CO)
- The change in pressure (ΔP) is mean arterial pressure (MAP) minus central venous pressure (CVP)
- Resistance (R) is TPR

Hence:

$$CO = \frac{MAP\text{-}CVP}{TPR}$$

Cardiac output can be increased by increasing contractility (to generate higher MAP) or heart rate, but the main mechanism of regulation is via changes in peripheral vascular tone (i.e. TPR) as explained by Poiseulle's equation. Changes in arteriolar diameter are the main mechanism of controlling local blood flow.

Poiseuille's equation

This law relates to the influence of fluid viscosity (η), the length of tube (L) and its radius (r) on resistance:

$$R = \frac{8\eta L}{\pi r^4}$$

Substituting in the previous resistance equation gives:

$$Q = \frac{\Delta P}{L} \cdot \frac{\pi r^4}{8\eta}$$

As blood viscosity and vessel length are relative constants, this simplifies to:

$$Q \propto \Delta P . r^4$$

In effect, this means:
- Most peripheral resistance is due to arterioles, because of the small diameter
- Blood flow increases linearly with blood pressure and to the fourth power of vessel radius
- Therefore, very small changes in vessel radius profoundly affect resistance, e.g. doubling the radius increases flow 16-fold

Poiseuille's equation also defines how an increase in blood viscosity increases resistance and blood pressure.

Flow velocity

Flow velocity is the velocity of blood in centimetres per second in a vessel or group of vessels. Unlike the overall volumetric flow (measured in

> ## Clinical insight
>
> Anemia – a reduction in erythrocytes – decreases blood viscosity and therefore blood pressure. Polycythemia has the opposite effect.

mL/min), flow velocity varies in different circulatory networks. It is inversely proportional to the cross-sectional area of the network (**Table 1.14**). The combined cross-sectional area of capillaries is very large. Consequently, slow capillary flow (<0.1 cm/s) allows time for exchange of nutrients, gases and waste between blood and cells.

Laminar and turbulent flow

Blood flow is normally laminar, i.e. concentric layers of fluid move parallel to the axis of the vessel (**Figure 1.33**). Vessel wall friction creates a gradient of velocity, with slower flow closer to the wall.

Turbulent, or disturbed, flow may occur if:
- Velocity increases as it goes through narrower spaces
- Viscosity reduces
- Vessel diameter increases.

Turbulent flow requires more pressure to achieve a given flow rate and is less efficient.

Blood pressure

Blood pressure is the force that blood exerts on vascular walls. It is measured in mil-

> ### Guiding principle
> 1 mmHg = 133.3 pascals (Pa)

limeters of mercury (mmHg), i.e. the number of millimeters by which it can raise a column of mercury in a manometer. In this section, blood pressure refers to systemic blood pressure, routinely measured with a sphygmomanometer at the brachial artery (see page 120).

Vessels	Cross-sectional area (cm²)	Flow velocity (cm/s)
Aorta	4	40
Capillaries	5000	<0.1
IVC and SVC	14	15

Table 1.14 Cross sectional area and flow velocity in the aorta, capillaries and vena cavae. IVC, inferior vena cava; SVC, superior vena cava.

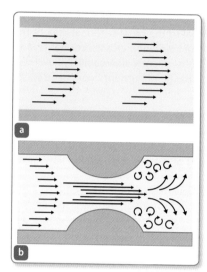

Figure 1.33 Flow through blood vessels. (a) Laminar flow. Friction between the vessel wall and flowing blood causes a parabolic velocity profile with the highest flow velocity centrally and the slowest at the periphery. (b) Turbulent flow: acceleration through narrowed segment causes flow separation and vortex formation in the poststenosis region.

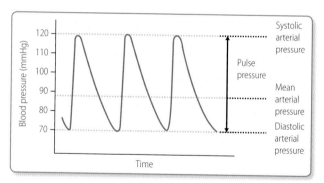

Figure 1.34 Systolic, diastolic and mean arterial blood pressure. The pulse pressure is the difference between the systolic pressure and the diastolic pressure.

Blood pressure is expressed as the systolic value over the diastolic value, for example 120/80 mmHg. Mean arterial pressure (MAP) is the average blood pressure over the period of the cardiac cycle (**Figure 1.34**).

Maximum blood pressure is reached during systole, and the minimum occurs in diastole. Although the heart is an intermittent pump, blood pressure is maintained during diastole by elastic recoil of the large arteries (**Figure 1.35**). Blood pressure declines the more distal a vessel is from the left ventricle, as flow energy is lost via friction and resistance decreases.

Determinants of blood pressure

Blood pressure is the sum of the arterial and venous pressures. However, central venous pressure (CVP) is usually discounted as it is close to zero (normally 2–5 mmHg). Recall the following relationship:

$$\text{Pressure } (P) = \text{flow } (Q) \times \text{resistance } (R)$$

Flow is equivalent to cardiac output and resistance equals TPR. Therefore:

$$\text{MAP} = \text{stroke volume} \times \text{heart rate} \times \text{TPR}$$

Guiding principle

Mean arterial blood pressure can be approximated by:

MAP = 1/3 systolic BP + 2/3 diastolic BP

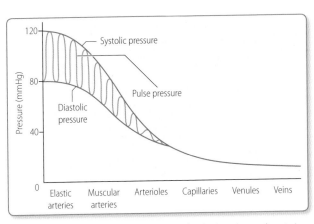

Figure 1.35 The first vessels in the arterial tree, the elastic and muscular arteries, transmit blood pressure with minimal loss. Through the arterioles there is a large fall in blood pressure and the pulse pressure falls until it is eventually lost.

This shows that an increase or a decrease in stroke volume, heart rate or TPR will cause a corresponding increase or decrease in MAP. As stroke volume is closely related to blood volume, the major determinants of MAP are:

- TPR
- Cardiac output (stroke volume × heart rate)
- Blood volume

Systolic blood pressure is mainly determined by stroke volume and arterial compliance. Diastolic blood pressure is mainly determined by TPR.

Control of blood pressure

Blood pressure is regulated in the short term by the cardiovascular center of the ANS (**Table 1.15**). TPR is also affected by blood vessel autoregulation (see page 51) and the influence of hormones and vasoactive chemicals. Long-term regulation is via hormonal control of blood volume and vascular tone.

Short-term control

The medullary cardiovascular center co-ordinates fast homeostatic mechanisms to ensure tissues have sufficient O_2, glucose and other essential metabolites (**Figure 1.36**).

Factor	Sympathetic activation	Parasympathetic activation
Heart rate	↑ (increasing CO)	↓
Contractility	↑ (increasing SV and CO)	-
Arterial vascular tone	↑ (increasing TPR)	↓
Venous tone	↑ (increasing CVP and CO)	↓
Hormone release	Adrenaline (epinephrine) from adrenal glands and renin from the kidneys	-
Blood pressure	↑	↓

Table 1.15 The ANS is central to global blood pressure control; CO, cardiac output; SV, stroke volume; TPR, total peripheral resistance. CVP, central venous pressure.

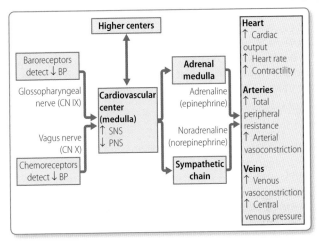

Figure 1.36 Short-term mechanisms of blood pressure control. A decrease in blood pressure is detected by baroreceptors and chemoreceptors. The cardiovascular center coordinates the response through activation of the sympathetic nervous system (SNS) and inhibition of the parasympathetic nervous system (PNS) to cause a compensatory increase in blood pressure.

Baroreceptors Stretch receptors of the aortic arch and carotid sinus send signals to the cardiovascular center via cranial nerves IX and X. An

Clinical insight

In essential hypertension (see page 185), the baroreflex threshold is reset to a higher point.

increase in the rate of baroreceptor action potential firing stimulates the PNS, and inhibits the SNS, to decrease blood pressure. A decrease in pressure has the opposite effect. This baroreflex system is rapid and modifiable (e.g. to accommodate exercise) but doesn't affect long-term control.

Chemoreceptors Chemoreceptors of the aortic arch and carotid bodies are sensitive to changes in blood O_2, CO_2 and pH. Their signals also travel in the IX and X cranial nerves to the medulla. They have a greater effect on the respiratory than the cardiovascular center.

Chemoreceptors are activated by decreased O_2 and pH and increased CO_2, and cause an increase in vascular tone and *decrease* in heart rate. The bradycardic effect is concurrently overridden by sympathetic stimulation due to lung stretch receptor activation, so that the overall effect is an increase in heart rate, vascular tone and blood pressure.

Muscle receptors Muscle chemo- and stretch receptors activate the SNS during activity.

Influence of higher brain regions Higher brain regions can influence blood pressure homeostasis. For example, the amygdala and hypothalamus stimulate the fight-or-flight response to a perceived threat:
- Increased blood pressure, heart rate, breathing rate
- Pupil dilation
- Decreased digestion
- Diversion of blood to skeletal muscles
- Release of stored energy.

> **Clinical insight**
>
> Chronic stress can increase risk of CHD, via increases in blood pressure, triglycerides and cholesterol leading to atherosclerosis.

Hormones Short-term regulation of blood pressure is also influenced by the hormones adrenaline (epinephrine), angiotensin II (AT II), antidiuretic hormone (ADH) and atrial natriuretic peptide (ANP) (**Table 1.16**). The latter three are also important in long-term blood pressure regulation.

Long-term control

Long-term blood pressure regulation is largely via control of blood volume. This is modified by systems of Na^+ and water reabsorption and excretion in the renal tubules (**Figure 1.37**).

Antidiuretic hormone Osmoreceptors in the hypothalamus sense fluctuations in serum osmolality, i.e. in how concentrated plasma is with electrolytes (particularly Na^+). An increase in osmolality results in ADH secretion via the posterior pituitary. ADH causes:

Hormone	Source	Stimulant	Action
Adrenaline (epinephrine)	Adrenal medulla	SNS	Nonselective adrenoreceptor agonist – similar to noradrenaline (norepinephrine) action
Angiotensin II	Liver	Hypotension	Vasoconstricion, renal water and salt retention
Antidiuretic hormone	Hypothalamus/ posterior pituitary gland		
Atrial natriuretic peptide	Atrial myocardium	Atrial stretch	Vasodilation, and augments renal salt and water clearance

Table 1.16 Hormones influencing blood pressure. SNS, sympathetic nervous system

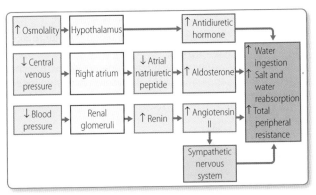

Figure 1.37 Long-term blood pressure regulation through control of blood volume. The overall effect is a reflex increase in blood pressure by increasing both blood volume and total peripheral resistance.

- Peripheral vasoconstriction
- Thirst
- Increased aquaporin expression in cells of the distal renal tubule and collecting dust, resulting in increased water reabsorption.

> ## Clinical insight
>
> A low salt diet is advised for hypertensive patients as Na⁺ is the main contributor to plasma osmolality, and increases blood volume

This dilutes blood, and increases TPR and blood volume and therefore blood pressure.

Atrial natriuretic peptide Atrial myocardial cells release ANP in response to stretch, i.e. increased blood volume or venous return. ANP causes:

- Peripheral vasodilation
- Dilation of afferent and constriction of efferent glomerular arterioles to increase glomerular filtration rate (GFR)
- Reduced renal Na⁺ and water reabsorption
- Inhibition of the renin–angiotensin–aldosterone system (RAAS).

This decreases both TPR and blood volume, and therefore blood pressure.

Renin–angiotensin–aldosterone system (RAAS) RAAS is a hormonal cascade that increases TPR and blood volume to raise blood pressure (**Figure 1.38**).

Renin is an enzyme produced by granular cells of the renal juxtaglomerular apparatus (JGA). Release is stimulated by:

- Decrease in arterial blood pressure – detected by JGA

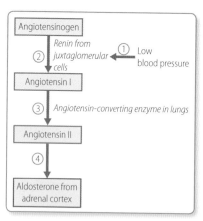

Figure 1.38 The renin–angiotensin–aldosterone cascade. (1), Renin is released from the juxtaglomerular cells in response to low blood pressure. (2), Renin cleaves angiotensinogen into angiotensin I. (3), Angiotensin I is converted into angiotensin II by angiotensin-converting enzyme. (4), Angiotensin II stimulates aldosterone release from the adrenal cortex.

- Low Na^+ detected in the ultrafiltrate – detected by macula densa of JGA
- SNS stimulation to the JGA.

Renin converts plasma angiotensinogen produced by liver cells into angiotensin (AT). AT is subsequently converted by angiotensin-converting enzyme (ACE) into AT II. AT II causes:

- Powerful vasoconstriction
- Increase in renal Na^+ and water reabsorption
- SNS stimulation
- Aldosterone release
- ADH release.

Aldosterone is a mineralo-corticoid hormone that, like ADH, increases renal Na^+ and water reabsorption at the DCT and collecting ducts.

> **Clinical insight**
>
> Angiotensin converting enzyme (ACE) inhibitors and angiotensin II receptor blockers (ARBs) are two antihypertensive drugs that block RAAS activation

Hemostasis

Blood is a water-based fluid that distributes metabolic nutrients, gases and waste products as well as blood cells and many proteins (**Table 1.17**).

Hemostasis is a sequence of events that prevents blood loss from damaged vessels and is the start of wound healing. It has three stages:

1. Vasoconstriction
2. Platelet aggregation forming a 'platelet plug'
3. The coagulation cascade forming a fibrin clot.

The end result is a thrombus; a collection of platelets, dead (predominately red) cells and a matrix of the protein fibrin. Platelet aggregation is quicker but weaker than the fibrin deposition of the cascade and is of greater importance in high-flow, arterial vessels – forming paler, platelet-rich 'white clots'. Fibrin deposition occurs more in low-flow venous vessels, resulting in fibrin and erythrocyte-rich 'red clots'.

Vasoconstriction

Injury to a blood vessel results in vasoconstriction to limit blood loss. Constriction is triggered by:

Blood composition			Example	Function
55% plasma	92% water		-	Solvent
	8% dissolved substances	Nutrients	Glucose	Energy metabolism
		Respiratory gases	O_2, CO_2	Cellular respiration
		Proteins	Albumin	Transport of substances, maintain intravascular oncotic pressure
			Clotting factors	Blood clotting
			Immuno-globulins	Adaptive immune response
		Lipids		Cell membranes, energy, hormones
		Electrolytes	Na^+, K^+, Ca^{2+}, Cl^-	Membrane potentials and transport
			H^+, HCO_3^-	Body fluid acidity
44% red blood cells (erythrocytes)				O_2 transport
1% white blood cells (leukocytes)				Immune

Table 1.17 Blood constituents and their functions.

Clinical insight

Thromboembolism is when a piece of a thrombus breaks off and embolizes (i.e. travels) downstream to partially or completely occlude a vessel. Deep vein venous thromboembolism is the most common, and can result in pulmonary embolism.

- A direct vascular smooth muscle cell response
- Endothelial cell release of vasoconstrictive mediators
- Local pain reflexes.

Platelet aggregation

Platelets are anuclear fragments of megakaryocytes produced in the bone marrow. They are continually produced and last for 10–12 days. Platelets contain vesicles (granules):

- α-granules: clotting factors, inflammatory mediators and growth factors

- Dense granules: ATP, ADP, serotonin (a potent vasoconstrictor) and Ca^{2+}
- Lysosymes

A number of platelet agonists trigger specific pathways of platelet activation, resulting in activation of the GPIIb/IIIa complex. Platelet aggregation is initiated by exposure to subendothelial components in the extracellular matrix (ECM). von Willebrand factor (vWF), a circulating protein, binds to both ECM collagen and to platelet surface glycoprotein GpIb (**Figure 1.39**). This results in translocation of glycoprotein complex IIb/IIIa (GpIIb/ IIIa) to the platelet surface. Platelets aggregate by bonding via GpIIb/IIIa complexes.

Platelet activation

Platelets are activated to release their secretory vesicles (i.e. degranulate) by:

- Adenosine diphosphate (ADP)
- Thrombin, an enzyme of the coagulation system
- Calcium
- Thromboxane A_2, a lipid signalling molecule.

Degranulation promotes aggregation, further platelet activation, the coagulation cascade and inflammation. Conversely,

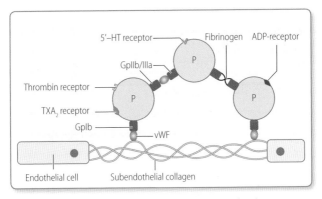

Figure 1.39 Platelets constitutively express GpIb on their surface, but once activated they express GpIIb/ IIIa, which mediates strong bonds between them. Gp, glycoprotein; P, platelet; TXA_2, thromboxane; vWF, von Willebrand factor.

prostacyclin release by endothelial cells and leukocytes inhibits platelet aggregation and their release from the bone marrow.

The coagulation cascade

The coagulation cascade is a series of amplifying reactions of clotting factors resulting in fibrin clot formation (**Figure 1.40**). Clotting factors are soluble pro-enzymes (e.g. factor X or FX) present in circulation that are cleaved to become active enzymes (e.g. FXa).

The reactions of the coagulation system often take place on the surface of platelets and require Ca^{2+} as a co-factor. The cascade can be initiated by endothelial damage (the extrinsic pathway) or intrinsic to ongoing hemostasis (the intrinsic pathway).

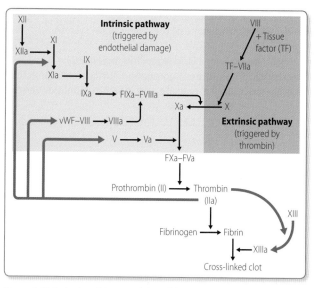

Figure 1.40 Activation of the coagulation of clotting cascade occurs via the extrinsic or intrinsic pathways, but both converge on generation of thrombin, which forms an insoluble fibrin mesh.

The extrinsic pathway

Endothelial damage exposes tissue factor (TF), which binds factor VII (FVII), activating factor VII to FVIIa–TF. This complex activates FX, which associates with its co-factor, FV, to form FXa–FVa (a small amount of active FV is present spontaneously). FXa–FVa converts prothrombin (FII) into thrombin (FIIa), which cleaves soluble, circulating fibrinogen – the soluble precursor of fibrin – into insoluble fibrin. Only a small clot is formed, but the intrinsic pathway is activated to form a full fibrin clot.

> ### Guiding principle
> Clotting factors are synthesized by the liver and have a short half-life. FII, FVII, FIX, and FX require vitamin K for their synthesis.

Thrombin produced by the extrinsic pathway activates:

- FV
- FVIII (by cleavage from circulating FVII–vWF complexes)
- FXI
- Platelets

The extrinsic pathway is rapidly terminated by the extrinsic pathway inhibitor (EPI) that blocks activation of FX by FVIIa–TF.

The intrinsic pathway

This is triggered by thrombin generated by the extrinsic pathway or from platelet degranulation. FIXa–FVIIIa complexes activate FX, which is able to generate large amounts of thrombin and therefore a fibrin clot.

Thrombolysis

Thrombolysis (or fibrinolysis) is the process of cleaving insoluble fibrin into soluble degradation products, to remove clots (**Figure 1.41**). This limits thrombus size, allows remodeling and breaks the thrombus down once the causative damage has been repaired.

Cleavage is mediated by plasmin, which circulates as inactive plasminogen and is activated by tissue plasminogen activator (tPA). Endothelial cells release tPA in response to the presence of thrombin.

Figure 1.41 Mechanism of thrombolysis: plasmin breaks down insoluble fibrin into soluble degradation products. tPA, tissue plasminogen activator.

Anti-coagulation systems

The body has several systems to prevent unnecessary activation of the coagulation cascade:

- Antithrombins (e.g. antithrombin III) inhibit thrombin and other active clotting factors, blocking progression of the cascade
- Heparin works by activating antithrombin III, making it rapidly effective
- The protein C system. In response to the presence of thrombin, thrombomodulin is expressed on the surface of intact endothelial cells. Circulating protein C and its co-factor protein S bind to thrombomodulin and break down FVa and FVIIIa.

> **Clinical insight**
>
> Synthetic ('recombinant') tPA is used to promote thrombolysis and reopen blocked vessels in cases of ischemic stroke and myocardial infarction.

Lipid metabolism

Lipid molecules contain carbon, hydrogen and oxygen, and principally consist of non-polar carbon–hydrogen (C–H) bonds. They are consumed in the diet and synthesized *de novo*. Lipids can be hydrolyzed to yield fatty acids or complex alcohols, which are important energy fuels for cellular metabolism.

They are a diverse group of substances with diverse chemical structures and functions (**Table 1.18**).

> **Clinical insight**
>
> Warfarin is an anticoagulant that antagonizes the effects of vitamin K, preventing the formation of clotting factors (II, VII, IX and X). Its onset is much slower (2–3 days) than heparin anticoagulation (<12 hours). Over-anticoagulation can cause spontaneous bleeding with serious clinical consequences

Function	Examples	Structure
Principle component of biological membranes	Glycerophospholipids	Derivatives of phosphatidic acid
	Sphingolipids	Derivatives of the amino acid sphingosine
Hormones	Prostaglandins	Fatty acid (mostly arachidonic acid) derivatives
	Steroids	Cholesterol based
Energy storage	Acylglycerols	Glycerol backbone with fatty acid attached
Energy metabolite	Fatty acids	12–20 carbon hydrocarbons with COOH group. Saturated have no double bonds
Vitamins	Terpenes, e.g. vitamins A, E and K	Polymer of 5 carbon isoprene
Transport of lipophilic compounds	Lipoproteins	Protein-emulsified lipid assemblies

Table 1.18 Lipid functions. COOH, carboxylic acid.

Polarity
Lipids have a hydrophobic tail group which is non-polar, and makes them soluble in organic solvents and insoluble in water. Some lipids also contain other polar groups that make them amphiphilic (amphipathic), i.e. they have both polar, soluble, water-loving (hydrophilic) and non-polar, fat-loving (lipophilic) properties. Amphiphilic lipids have important biological functions, for example phospholipids constitute the lipid bilayer structure of cell membranes.

Lipolysis
Lipids are hydrolyzed to fatty acids and glycerol in adipose and muscle tissues when energy is required.

Guiding principle
Carbon–carbon double bonds:
- Saturated fatty acids – 0
- Monounsaturated fatty acids – 1
- Polyunsaturated fatty acids > 1.

1. Triglyceride hydrolysis   Fasting, exercise or stress stimulates triglyceride hydrolysis by lipase. Glycerol is then phosphorylated to glycerol 3-phosphate before being oxidized to dihydroxyacetone phosphate. Glyceraldehyde-3-phosphate can be converted to either pyruvate or glucose in the liver.

2. Fatty acid co-linkage to coenzyme A   Fatty acids are first activated in the cytosol when they are bound by a coenzyme A (CoA). This is catalyzed by acyl CoA synthetase and is irreversible.

Step 1: fatty acid + ATP → acyl adenylate + pyrophosphate
Step 2: acyl adenylate + CoASH → acyl CoA + AMP

A thioester bond is formed between the fatty acid carboxyl group and the sulfhydryl group of CoA.

3. The carnitine shuttle   Acyl CoA can only enter mitochondria via the carnitine shuttle. Carnitine is a nitrogenous cation that binds to acyl CoA to form acylcarnitine. This is able to cross the outer and inner mitochondrial membranes in exchange for unbound carnithine moving out of mitochondria. This is the rate-limiting step in fatty acid oxidation.

Regulation of lipolysis

Lipolysis is regulated through the control of lipase activity (**Figure 1.42**). Counter-regulatory hormones stimulate lipase when energy reserves are low: adrenaline (epinephrine), noradrenaline (norepinephrine), growth hormone, cortisol and glucagon. Conversely, insulin inhibits lipase.

Fatty acid oxidation

Fatty acids are oxidized by β-oxidation in mitochondria and peroxisomes to generate acetyl CoA, NADH and $FADH_2$. Acetyl-CoA enters the citric acid cycle and the latter act as oxidizing co-factors in the electron transport chain. Each $FADH_2$ and NADH generates two and three molecules of ATP, respectively.
Before oxidation, unsaturated fatty acids must have their double bonds broken by isomerase and reductase enzymes.

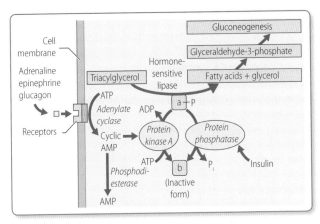

Figure 1.42 Regulation of lipase activity.

Glycerol

Glycerol is a 3-carbon polyol (sugar alcohol) with three hydroxyl groups, and is the backbone of all triglyceride lipids. Once converted to glyceraldehyde-3-phosphate, it can enter glycolysis or gluconeogenesis in the liver. Alternatively, it can be used as a substrate for triacylglycerol or phospholipid synthesis in the liver and adipose tissue.

> ### Guiding principle
>
> Peroxisomes are small organelles that breakdown very long chain and branched chain fatty acids, polyamines, amino acids and synthesize plasmalogens. Peroxisomal oxidation is stimulated by a fat-rich meal or some lipid-lowering drugs such as fibrates.

Lipogenesis

Fatty acids synthesis is the production of palmitic acid from acetyl CoA and malonyl CoA. It occurs in the liver, lactating mammary glands and adipose tissue if dietary intake is insufficient. There are four stages, the later three occurring in the cytosol:
1. Acetyl CoA synthesis and the citrate shuttle
2. Malonyl CoA synthesis
3. Formation of malonyl transferase
4. The fatty acid elongation cycle.

Palmitic acid is a 16-carbon fatty acid and the most abundant in the body. It is the starting point for all fatty acids. It normally exists dissociated from its H^+ ion as palmitate ion.

Acetyl coenzyme A synthesis

Acetyl CoA is synthesized from pyruvate by pyruvate dehydrogenase and by mitochondrial β-oxidation of fatty acids.

The citrate shuttle   Acetyl CoA is transported from mitochondria to the cytosol as citrate:

1. Acetyl CoA reacts with oxaloacetate to form citrate
2. Tricarboxylate translocase transports citrate to the cytosol
3. Citrate is cleaved back to oxaloacetate and acetyl CoA in the cytosol by an ATP-dependent enzyme called ATP-citrate lyase.

This requires 14 NADPH as reducing agents, and produces 8 for every molecule of palmitate produced. The pentose phosphate pathway provides the deficit.

Malonyl coenzyme A synthesis

Some acetyl CoA is carboxylated to form malonyl CoA in an irreversible two-step reaction that requires bicarbonate, biotin and ATP. It is a commitment step in fatty acid synthesis, as malonyl CoA is only involved in fatty acid synthesis.

Both steps are catalyzed by acetyl CoA carboxylase:

- Acetyl CoA is converted to carboxybiotin; one ATP is used
- The carboxyl group is transferred from the biotin to the acetyl CoA to form malonyl CoA.

This is the key regulatory step for fatty acid synthesis (see page 74). The 'extra' carbon of malonyl CoA is what allows lipogenesis to be thermodynamically possible.

Fatty acid synthase

Fatty acid synthase is a dimeric, 7-enzyme complex that synthesizes palmitic acid from either acyl CoA or malonyl CoA. Each domain is responsible for different steps of synthesis (**Table 1.19**).

Firstly, acetyl CoA or malonyl CoA attach to an oxygen atom of acetyl transferase or malonyl transferase, respectively. Acetyl groups are transferred to the condensing enzyme β-ketoacyl

Domain	Enzymes/proteins	Function
1. Condensing unit	Acetyl transferase	Substrate binding
	Malonyl transferase	
	β-ketoacyl ACP synthase	Decarboxylation – liberation of CO_2; condensation ('merging') of acetyl and malonyl groups to form acetoacetyl-ACP
2. Reduction unit	ACP	Binds acetoacetyl group
	β-keto - acylreductase	Reduces acetoacetyl-ACP to β-hydroxybutyryl-ACP
	β-hydroxybutyryl-ACP dehydratase	Dehydrates β-hydroxybutyryl-ACP to trans-Δ^2-butenoyl-ACP (with a double bond)
	Enoyl reductase	Reduces trans-Δ^2-butenoyl-ACP to remove double bond and form butyryl-ACP
3. Palmitate release unit	Thioesterase	Releases palmitic acid via hydrolysis

Table 1.19 The three domains of the fatty acid synthase complex and their functions. ACP, acetyl carrier protein.

synthase. Malonyl groups are then transferred to the acyl carrier protein.

The two carbons of the malonyl group attached to the acyl carrier protein are elongated by a cycle of condensation and reduction reactions to form 16-carbon palmitoyl. Finally, this is hydrolyzed to palmitate. The stoichiometry can be summarized as:

$$8 \text{ acetyl CoA} + 7 \text{ ATP} + 14 \text{ NADPH} + 6 \text{ H}^+$$
$$\downarrow$$
$$\text{Palmitate} + 14 \text{ NADP}^+ + 8 \text{ CoA} + 6 \text{ H}_2\text{O} + 7 \text{ ADP} + 7 \text{ P}_i$$

Guiding principle

Biotin is a water-soluble B vitamin (B7) and important for carboxylase catalyzed reactions.

Further elongation

Longer fatty acids are synthesized by microsomes – vesicles of budded endoplasmic reticulum. Two carbon units are added to the carbonyl end of saturated and unsaturated fatty acids. Solubility rapidly decreases as chain length increases.

Unsaturation of fatty acids

Microsomal enzymes also add double bonds to unsaturate long chain acyl CoAs, such as cnverting stearoyl CoA to oleoyl CoA. An oxidase enzyme introduces a cis-Δ^9 double bond, and requires O_2 and NADH, and releases two molecules of water.

> ### Guiding principle
>
> Double bonds in unsaturated fatty acids increase solubility and lower melting point. This underlies the fluidity of cell membranes.

> ### Clinical insight
>
> Fibric acid derivatives (fibrates) are used as drugs to lower triglyceride concentration. They:
>
> - Induce gene expression of lipolytic enzymes such as lipoprotein lipase
> - Decrease the expression of apolipoprotein C3, a protein that inhibits lipoprotein lipase
> - Promote a shift toward larger, more buoyant low-density lipoprotein (LDL) particles that are less susceptible to oxidation and have increased affinity for the LDL receptor

Regulation of fatty acid metabolism

Fatty acid metabolism is predominately regulated by hormones that affect acetyl CoA carboxylase activity (**Figure 1.43**):

- When energy is required, adrenaline (epinephrine) and glucagon inactivate it via phosphorylation by AMP protein kinase
- When energy is not required, insulin activates it via dephosphorylation by phosphatase 2A.

Acetyl CoA carboxylase is also activated by citrate and inhibited by AMP and palmitoyl CoA.

Lipogenesis is tightly coordinated with fatty acid breakdown, i.e. β-oxidation (**Table 1.20**).

Prostaglandins

Arachidonate is a 20-carbon polyunsaturated fatty acid derived from linoleate. It is the starting point for the basis of the prostaglandins: prostacyclins, thromboxanes and leukotrienes

Figure 1.43 Regulation of acetyl coenzyme A carboxylase activity. +, activates; P, phosphate; Pi, inorganic phosphate.

Feature	Synthesis	Oxidation
Intracellular location	Cytoplasm	Mitochondria
Initial substrates	Acetyl CoA or malonyl CoA	Fatty acyl CoA
Thioester linkage of intermediates	Protein-SH (acyl carrier protein)	CoA
Coenzymes	NADPH	FAD$^+$ and NAD$^+$
Bicarbonate dependence	Yes	No
Energy state favoring process	High ATP	High ADP
Citrate activation	Yes	No
Acyl CoA inhibition	Yes	No
Highest activity	Fed	Fasting or starvation

Table 1.20 Comparison of fatty acid synthesis and breakdown (β-oxidation). ATP, adenosine triphosphate; CoA, coenzyme A; CoASH, Acetyl coenzyme A; FAD$^+$, flavin adenine dinucleotide (oxidized form); NAD$^+$, nicotinamide adenine dinucleotide (oxidized form); NADPH, nicotinamide adenine dinucleotide phosphate (reduced form).

(**Figure 1.44**). These locally acting hormones have a short half-life but have vital functions, including:

- Stimulating the inflammatory response
- Regulating local blood flow

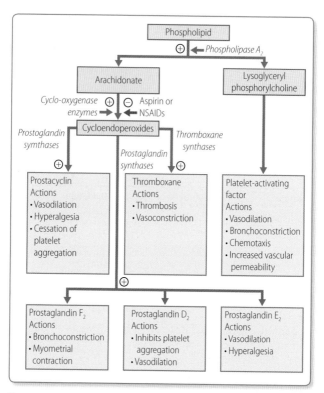

Figure 1.44 Prostaglandin biosynthesis and their actions. +, activates; –, inhibits; NSAID, non-steroidal anti-inflammatory drug.

- Modulating ion transport across membranes
- Propagating synaptic transmission
- Sleep induction.

Cholesterol metabolism

Cholesterol is a 27-carbon steroid alcohol (sterol) lipid (**Figure 1.45**). It is a key component of cell membranes, allowing their fluid movement, and is the precursor to vitamin D, bile acids and steroid hormones, including testosterone and cortisol.

Figure 1.45 Cholesterol.

Cholesterol is consumed in the diet and synthesized de novo in the liver and intestine. On average, 800 mg of cholesterol is synthesized daily in a person on a low-cholesterol diet.

Cholesterol synthesis

Cholesterol biosynthesis begins with formation of isopentenyl pyrophosphate from acetyl CoA (**Figure 1.46**). The first step is the condensation of acetyl CoA with acetoacetyl CoA, forming 3-hydroxy-3-methylglutaryl CoA (HMG-CoA), a reaction catalyzed by HMG CoA synthase.

Formation of mevalonate HMG-CoA, which is present in the cytosol and mitochondria of the liver, is reduced to mevalonate by HMG-CoA reductase. This reaction requires NADPH. This is the first irreversible, committed step of cholesterol synthesis. Mevalonate is then converted to iso-pentenyl pyrophosphate in a series of three ATP-dependent reactions.

Synthesis of squalene The second stage of cholesterol synthesis is the synthesis of squalene, a 30-carbon hydrocarbon molecule, from five five-carbon molecules of

> ## Clinical insight
>
> Aspirin (acetylsalicylate) decreases inflammation by inhibiting the activity of prostaglandin synthase. It irreversibly inhibits the cyclo-oxygenase activity of this enzyme by acetylating the serine hydroxyl group. It is also an antithrombotic agent, because it blocks the production of prostaglandin A_2, a potent aggregator of blood platelets.

> ## Clinical insight
>
> Statins lower blood cholesterol by inhibiting HMG - CoA reductase, the rate-limiting enzyme of cholesterol biosynthesis.

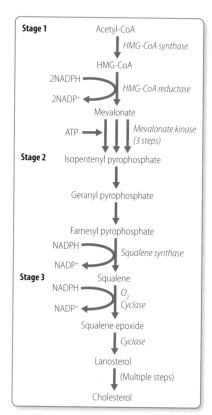

Figure 1.46 Biosynthesis of cholesterol. HMG-CoA, 3-hydroxy-3-methylglutaryl CoA. NADPH, nicotinamide adenine dinucleotide phosphate; ATP, adenosine triphosphate.

isopentenyl pyrophosphate. This process starts with the isomerization of isopentenyl pyrophosphate to form dimethylallyl pyrophosphate.

Formation of squalene epoxide The third stage is the cyclization of squalene to form squalene epoxide. This requires O_2 and NADPH. Squalene epoxide then undergoes cyclization to lanosterol in a reaction catalyzed by cyclase. Lanosterol is then converted to cholesterol, a 27-carbon molecule, by the removal of three methyl groups and the reduction of a double bond by NADPH.

Regulation of cholesterol synthesis Cholesterol synthesis is regulated by mechanisms that sense the cellular level of cholesterol and modify HMG CoA reductase levels and activity:

- Sterol regulatory element: a transcription factor that inhibits enzyme gene expression in the presence of sterols
- Non-sterol metabolites: derivatives of mevalonate inhibit enzyme gene expression
- AMP-activated protein kinase: phosphorylates and decreases enzyme activity when ATP levels are low
- Enzyme degradation is also tightly regulated.

Cholesterol absorption

Cholesterol esters in the gut are hydrolyzed by cholesterol esterases, secreted by the pancreas and small intestine, to free cholesterol. Cholesterol must be emulsified to be absorbed: conjugated bile acids form micelles with free cholesterol, fatty acids, monoglycerides, and phospholipids.

Most cholesterol is absorbed in the middle jejunum and terminal ileum through the transmembrane transporter protein Niemann–Pick C1-like 1 protein. 30–60% of dietary cholesterol is absorbed daily. Once absorbed into the intestinal mucosa cell, it is packaged into large lipoproteins called chylomicrons.

> **Clinical insight**
>
> Ezetimibe is a potent cholesterol-lowering drug that works by blocking cholesterol absorption mediated by the Niemann–Pick C1-like 1 protein.

Cholesterol esterification

As free cholesterol is cytotoxic, it is esterified in the liver to cholesterol ester by acyl cholesterol acyl transferase. Cholesterol esters are stored in intracellular lipid drops and constitute 70% of plasma cholesterol.

> **Clinical insight**
>
> Familial hypercholesterolemia is an inherited condition causing high blood cholesterol concentrations. There are heterozygous and homozygous forms, affecting 1 in 500 and 1 in 1,000,000 of the UK population, respectively.

Esterification requires energy-dependent activation of a fatty acid with CoA to form an acyl CoA. The acyl CoA reacts with a hydroxyl group on cholesterol to form an ester.

Lipoprotein esterification Esterification also occurs in the blood, in lipoproteins, the lipid transport vesicles. This is catalyzed by lecithin-cholesterol acyl transferase and does not require CoA; instead a fatty acid is transferred from lecithin. The enzyme is activated by apolipoprotein A-I, the major apolipoprotein in high density lipoprotein (HDL). Cholesterol esters are in the hydrophobic core of the lipoprotein molecule (**Table 1.21**).

Lipid absorption and transport: lipoproteins

Lipoproteins are spherical particles with non-polar neutral lipids in their core (i.e. triglycerides and cholesterol esters) and more polar amphipathic lipids (i.e. phospholipids and cholesterol) on their surface (**Figure 1.47**). They also have apolipoproteins on their surface, which bind lipids, cell receptors and act as co-factors for enzymes of lipid metabolism (**Table 1.22**).

Types

Lipoproteins are classified by their physiochemical properties (**Tables 1.21** and **1.23**). Generally, larger lipoproteins contain more core lipids, triglycerides and cholesterol esters, and less protein.

Pathways

Lipoprotein metabolism has four main pathways with discrete functions in lipid transport.

Class	Cholesterol (%)	Phospholipids (%)	Apolipoproteins (%)	Triglycerides (%)	Cholesterol ester (%)
CM	2	7	2	86	3
VLDL	7	18	8	55	12
IDL	9	19	19	23	29
LDL	8	22	22	6	42
HDL-2	5	33	40	5	17
HDL-3	4	25	55	3	13

Table 1.21 Chemical composition of lipoproteins. CM, chylomicron; VLDL, very low density lipoprotein; IDL, intermediate density lipoprotein; LDL, low density lipoprotein; HDL, high density lipoprotein.

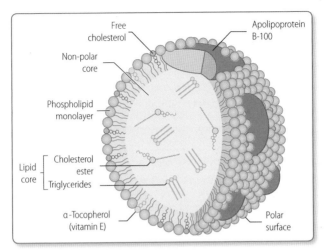

Figure 1.47 Lipoprotein structure.

1. The exogenous pathway
2. The endogenous pathway
3. Intracellular cholesterol transport
4. Reverse cholesterol transport.

The exogenous pathway

The exogenous lipoprotein pathway transports lipids absorbed by the intestine to the liver and peripheral cells (**Figure 1.48**).

- Chylomicrons are assembled in the endoplasmic reticulum of endocytes by combining triglycerides with apolipoprotein B-48
- They are secreted into the circulation, where they acquire additional lipoproteins (e.g. apolipoproteins E and CIIII) from HDL
- Apolipoprotein C-II activates lipoprotein lipase on the luminal surface of endothelial cells, which hydrolyzes chylomicrons to free fatty acids
- The free fatty acids are either taken up by adipose tissue and stored as triglycerides or taken up by muscle and used as an energy source.

Apolipoprotein	Function	Lipoprotein carrier
A-I	Co-factor for cholesteryl ester transfer protein	CM, HDL
A-II	Unknown	HDL
A-IV	Activates lecithin cholesterolacyltransferase Secretion of TG from liver binding protein to LDL receptor	CM, HDL
B-100	Secretion of TG from intestine	VLDL, IDL, LDL
B-48	Secretion of TG from liver binding protein to LDL receptor	CM
C-I	Activates lecithin cholesterolacyltransferase	CM, VLDL, HDL
C-II	Co-factor for lipoprotein lipase	CM, VLDL, HDL
C-III	Inhibits apo C-II Activates lipoprotein lipase	CM, VLDL, HDL
E	Facilitates uptake of CM and IDL remnants	CM, VLDL, HDL
(a)	Unknown	Lipoprotein (a)

Table 1.22 Functions of apolipoproteins. TG, triglyceride; CM, chylomicron; VLDL, very low density lipoprotein; IDL, intermediate density lipoprotein; LDL, low density lipoprotein; HDL, high density lipoprotein.

Remnant particles Chylomicrons are progressively hydrolyzed to chylomicron remnant particles. The surplus phospholipids and apolipoprotein A-I, are transferred back to HDL. Remnant particles are taken up by the liver through via hepatic apolipoprotein E and B-48 receptors. The triglycerides returned to the liver are used to power the biosynthetic activity of the liver, or they are repackaged with apolipoprotein B100 and secreted as very-low-density lipoprotein (VLDL) particles.

The endogenous pathway

This pathway transfers triglycerides synthesized by/transferred to the liver to peripheral cells for energy metabolism (**Figure 1.49**).

Variable	Chylomicron	VLDL	IDL	LDL	HDL	Lp(a)
Density (g/mL)	<0.95	0.95–1.006	1.006–1.019	1.019–1.063	1.063–1.210	1.040–1.130
Electrophoretic mobility	Origin	Pre-beta	Slow pre-beta	Beta	Alpha	Pre-beta
Molecular weight (Da)	$0.4–30 \times 10^9$	$5–10 \times 10^6$	$3.9–4.8 \times 10^6$	2.75×10^6	$1.8–3.6 \times 10^5$	$2.9–3.7 \times 10^6$
Diameter (nm)	>70	26–70	22–24	19–23	4–10	26–30
Lipid:lipoprotein ratio	99:1	90:10	85:15	80:20	50:50	75:26–64:36
Major lipids	Exogenous TG	Endogenous TG	Endogenous TG, CEs	CEs	PLs	CEs, PLs
Major proteins	A-I B-48 C-I C-II C-III	B-100 C-I C-II C-III E	B-100 E	B-100	A-I A-II	(a) B-100

Table 1.23 Properties of lipoproteins. CE, cholesterol ester; CM, chylomicrons; HDL, high-density lipoprotein; IDL, intermediate-density lipoprotein; LDL, lowdensity lipoprotein; Lp(a), lipoprotein(a); PL, phospholipid; TG, triglycerides; VLDL, very-low-density lipoprotein.

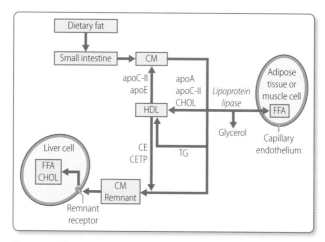

Figure 1.48 The exogenous lipoprotein pathway. apo, apolipoproteins; CE, cholesteryl ester; CETP; cholesterol ester transfer protein; CHOL; cholesterol; CM, chylomicrons; FFA, free fatty acids; HDL, high-density lipoprotein; IDL, intermediate-density lipoprotein; TG, triglycerides; VLDL, very-low-density lipoprotein.

Lipoproteins in the endogenous pathway contain apolipoprotein B-100, particularly VLDLs, which also contain apolipoprotein E and apolipoprotein C. The apolipoprotein C-II on the surface of VLDLs activates lipoprotein lipase on the surface of endothelial cells, which hydrolyze triglycerides to glycerol and fatty acids. The progressive hydrolysis of triglycerides in the core of a VLDL particle transforms it into intermediate density lipoprotein and eventually LDL.

About half of the apolipoprotein B100 particles in the exogenous pathway are removed by hepatic remnant receptors before undergoing complete hydrolysis. The remaining portion is converted to LDL. The triglyceride in LDL is further depleted by the cholesteryl-ester transfer protein, a plasma enzyme that removes triglycerides from LDL in exchange for cholesterol esters from HDL. During the transformation from VLDL to LDL, excess surface phospholipid and lipoproteins (except apolipoprotein B-100) are transferred to HDL.

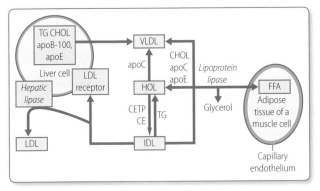

Figure 1.49 The endogenous lipoprotein pathway. apo, apolipoproteins; CE, cholesteryl ester; CETP; cholesteryl ester transfer protein; CHOL; cholesterol; CM, chylomicrons; FFA, free fatty acids; HDL, highdensity lipoprotein; IDL, intermediate-density lipoprotein; LDL, low-density lipoprotein; TG, triglycerides; VLDL, very-low-density lipoprotein.

Most LDL is returned to the liver through the LDL apolipo-protein B-100 receptor. The cholesterol can then be:
- Incorporated into lipoproteins
- Used in bile salt syntheses
- Excreted in bile.

Intracellular cholesterol transport

The intracellular transport of cholesterol is tightly regulated (**Figure 1.50**), as cholesterol affects membrane properties and is cytotoxic in excess.

Cellular cholesterol is derived from cellular synthesis, or through lipoprotein uptake via the LDL receptor. Receptor binding leads to lipoprotein endocytosis and lysosomal breakdown.

Apolipoproteins are degraded to small peptides and amino acids. Cholesterol esters are converted to free cholesterol by lysosomal acid lipase. Cholesterol is:
- Used for membrane biogenesis
- Stored in intracellular lipid drops after re-esterification
- Excreted in the reverse cholesterol transport pathway.

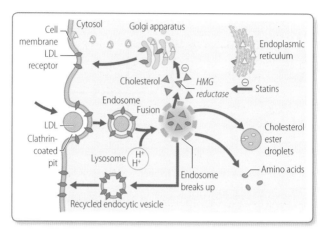

Figure 1.50 Overview of intracellular cholesterol transport. LDL, low-density lipoprotein. HMG CoA, 3-hydroxy-3-methylglutaryl CoA.

Regulation Excess intracellular cholesterol has a negative feedback effect on its own biosynthesis via HMG CoA reductase and LDL receptor down-regulation. It also induces the synthesis of proteins of the reverse cholesterol transport pathway.

Reverse cholesterol transport

This removes excess, potentially toxic, cellular cholesterol and transfers it to the liver for excretion (**Figure 1.51**). The main lipoprotein involved is HDL.

Cholesterol is actively pumped out of cells by the ATP-binding cassette transporter 1 (ABCA1) on to apolipoprotein A-I, which binds to cells to form nascent HDL.

Lecithin cholesterol acyl transferase is important in re-verse cholesterol transport, as esterification produces the more hydrophobic cholesterol esters that remain trapped in the HDL core, until they reach the liver.

> **Clinical insight**
>
> [LDL] (mmol/L) = [total cholesterol] − [HDL cholesterol] − ([triglyceride]/2.2)

Figure 1.51 The reverse cholesterol transport lipoprotein pathway. CE, cholesteryl ester; CETP, cholesteryl ester transfer protein; CHOL, cholesterol; CM, chylomicrons; FFA, free fatty acids; HDL, high-density lipoprotein; HTGL, hepatic triglyceride lipase; IDL, intermediate-density lipoprotein; LCAT, lecithin-cholesterol acyltransferase; TG, triglycerides; VLDL, very-low-density lipoprotein.

The liver selectively removes some of the cholesterol esters, to allow the lipid-depleted HDL to return to the circulation for further rounds of cholesterol removal.

The cholesteryl-ester transfer protein is also key, as it allows a large portion of cholesterol removed from HDL to transfer to LDL as cholesterol esters, which are then removed by hepatic LDL receptors.

Clinical insight

Increasing HDL ('good') cholesterol has been proposed as a way to reduce cardiovascular risk. HDL concentration is increased by exercise, taking nicotinic acid (vitamin B3), consuming alcohol in moderation, losing weight and stopping smoking.

Clinical essentials

The terms ischemic heart disease, coronary artery disease, atherosclerotic heart disease and coronary heart disease (CHD) are synonymous (in this book we use the latter). All are used to describe the condition whereby coronary arterial blood flow becomes restricted secondary to an accumulation of athero-sclerotic plaque. The resulting ischemia presents as angina, or as one of the acute coronary syndromes: unstable angina or myocardial infarction with or without ST elevation.

The clinical management of CHD centers on the recognition and treatment of signs and symptoms of atherosclerosis and cardiovascular risk factors including hypertension, hyperlipidemia, and arrhythmia, as discussed in Chapters 3–7. Complications include arrhythmias and heart failure (see Chapters 7 and 8).

Guidelines for diagnosis and management are continually changing, because there is such a large amount of research and a wide spectrum of diseases, including sub-clinical presentations.

Management depends largely on the stage of disease. Many people are at a stage early enough that primary and secondary prevention can have a significant effect with changes in lifestyle, exercise and diet, supplemented with drugs to lower risk factors and treat angina symptoms.

Treatment is graded from conservative to pharmacologic, then finally to surgical interventions if all else fails. CHD can be treated by all approaches at once, with a hybrid invasive and bypass strategy and medications to reduce the risk of graft and stent thrombosis. Structural heart diseases, such as aortic stenosis, are managed conservatively until surgical intervention is indicated.

2.1 History taking

The patient's history should produce a shortlist of potential diagnoses.

Symptoms

The key cardiovascular symptoms are chest pain, dyspnea, palpitations, ankle swelling and syncope.

Chest pain

Chest pain can be caused by benign, serious or life-threatening cardiac and non-cardiac conditions (**Table 2.1**).

Most cardiac chest pain (angina) is caused by myocardial ischemia due to atherosclerosis. It is less commonly caused by non-ischemic disease, including aortic dissection or pericarditis.

Character Angina is usually described by patients as a tight band around – or dull weight on, tightness of or discomfort in – the chest, making breathing difficult (**Figure 2.1**). It is usually brought on by exertion and relieved by rest. In contrast, non-cardiac chest pain is felt as a local sharpness (musculoskeletal pain), or diffuse burning (e.g. pain due to GERD). Aortic dissection is usually experienced as a tearing or gripping pain.

Like any pain, chest pain should be carefully characterized (**Table 2.2**) to differentiate the cause (**Table 2.3**).

Onset This can be:
- Sudden, spontaneous – aortic dissection, pneumothorax or massive pulmonary embolism
- Gradual, spontaneous – myocardial infarction
- Gradual, which increases during exertion – angina

Cause of chest pain	Percentage of presentations (%)
Musculoskeletal	36–45
Gastrointestinal conditions	8–19
Stable angina	10–12
Psychogenic	7.5–11.5
Acute cardiac ischemia	3
Pulmonary embolism	<1

Table 2.1 Causes of chest pain presentations in primary care.

Figure 2.1 Angina. (a) In Levine's sign, patients use a clenched fist in the center of their chest to describe the pain. Pointing with a single finger suggests a non-ischemic cause. (b) Pain is typically across the center of the chest and often radiates into the arms, neck and jaw.

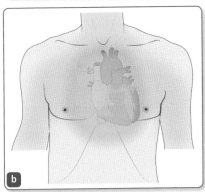

- Gradual, decreasing on exertion – normally due to musculoskeletal problems.

Radiation Cardiac pain radiates to the neck, jaw or shoulders/arms (typically left) as these areas share spinal nerves T1–T4 with afferents from the heart. Aortic dissection radiates to the back. Pain that radiates to the left axilla is usually non-cardiac (e.g. anxiety, pleural or musculoskeletal disease).

Characteristic	Example
Site	Central, unilateral, diffuse or focal?
Onset	Over minutes, hours, days or weeks?
Character	Sharp, dull, stabbing, heavy or constricting?
Radiation	Neck, jaw, back or arm?
Associated symptoms	Nausea, vomiting, dizziness, dyspnea or collapse?
Timing	Constant or intermittent?
Exacerbating and relieving factors	e.g. exertion or rest
Severity	Graded out of 10

Table 2.2 The SOCRATES mnemonic for characterizing pain.

Aspect of chest pain	GERD	Angina	Pericarditis	Pneumonia or PE
Site	Epigastric/retrosternal	Retrosternal, left pectoral region and the epigastrium	Central/left pectoral	Anywhere
Character	Burning	Crushing/aching	Sharp	Sharp
Radiation	Neck	Arms, neck, jaw	No	No
Associated symptoms	Waterbrash	Nausea, dyspnea, sweating	Fever	Shortness of breath, cough, fever
Exacerbating factors	Food, lying down	Exertion, cold, stress	Breathing, lying down	Breathing, coughing
Relieving factors	Milk, antacid	GTN, rest	NSAIDs, sitting forward	Holding breath

Table 2.3 Differentiating chest pain. GERD, gastroesophageal reflux disease; GTN, glyceryl trinitrate; NSAIDs, non-steroidal anti-inflammatory drugs; PE, pulmonary embolism.

Associated symptoms Acute severe chest pain is associated with tachycardia, sweating, nausea and vomiting.

> ## Clinical insight
> Chest pain that has been present constantly for years without complications is unlikely to be cardiac.

CHD pain often presents with symptoms of heart failure, including shortness of breath and ankle swelling.

Exacerbating/relieving factors Cardiac chest pain usually increases with myocardial oxygen demand; exercise, cold weather, consuming a large meal or stress. Chest pain that increases during rest or a specific movement is normally non-cardiac, such as anxiety or musculoskeletal causes.

Severity Rating pain on a scale of 0–10 helps to understand the patient's relative concept of their pain and to monitor changes.

Dyspnea

Dyspnea – shortness of breath – is the sensation of not being able to breathe enough. It often occurs with chest pain, but has non-cardiac causes (**Table 2.4**).

Types of breathlessness include:

- Orthopnea – breathlessness on lying supine; common in heart disease where alveolar fluid shifts with gravity to increase ventilation:perfusion mis-match when the patient lays supine.
- Paroxysmal nocturnal dyspnea – intermittent breathlessness which occurs during the night
- Tachypnea – increased respiratory rate of >20 breaths per minute.

Onset Defining the onset of breathlessness helps differentiate the cause and what action can be taken:

- One week after ceasing a diuretic indicates a medication review
- Sudden onset following a long-haul flight can suggest pulmonary embolus
- Intermittent breathlessness that coincides with palpitations suggests paroxysmal AF.

Type of feature	Angina	Asthma/COPD	Heart Failure	Pulmonary embolism	Pneumonia
Associated symptoms	Chest pain	Wheeze, cough	Fatigue	Pain, cough	Fever, cough
Exacerbating factors	Exertion	Allergens, aspirin	Supine	None	None
Relieving factors	Rest	β agonists	Diuretics	None	Oxygen
Risk factors	Hyper-tension, smoking	Occupation, smoking	Myocardial infarction	DVT, immobility	Malnutrition, immuno-suppression
Onset	Gradual	Acute	Gradual	Acute	Gradual

Table 2.4 Differentiating between causes of dyspnea. COPD, chronic obstructive pulmonary disease. DVT, deep vein thrombosis.

Associated symptoms Other symptoms experienced during dyspnea may include pain, wheeze or cough (**Table 2.5**).

Exacerbating factors Most breathlessness is worse on exertion and better at rest; the inverse suggests a psychological cause.

Severity Monitoring the severity of dyspnea helps gauge quality of life, and guide and monitor treatment (Table 8.2).

> **Clinical insight**
>
> Anxiety or allergens can exacerbate pre-existing breathlessness.

Palpitations

Palpitations are heartbeats that a person is aware of, and they have a variety of sensations and causes (**Table 2.6**). It is useful to ask the patient to tap the rhythm they feel and how long they feel it for (**Table 2.7**).

Most irregular rhythms are atrial fibrillation (AF), and most regular rhythms are sinus tachycardia, atrial flutter or supra-ventricular tachycardias (SVT).

Associated symptoms Breathlessness, chest pain and pre-syncope suggest serious underlying cardiac pathology.

Dyspnea symptom	Indicates	
Pain	On exertion indicates myocardial ischemia	
Wheeze	Cardiac asthma – pulmonary edema due to left ventricular failure	
Cough	White/frothy sputum	Pulmonary edema
	Pink/blood stained sputum	Mitral valve disease with pulmonary capillary rupture
		Infiltrative lung malignancy
	Gray/green/brown and purulent sputum	Infection
	Dry/non-productive/tickly	Side effect of angiotensin-converting enzyme inhibitors
		Asthma

Table 2.5 Symptoms associated with dyspnea and their cause.

Syncope

Syncope, or fainting, is a sudden and transient loss of consciousness with rapid recovery and no long-term consequences. It is caused by temporary global hypoperfusion of the brain due to hypotension. It can suggest serious cardiac pathology, pulmonary emboli, sepsis, or significant blood loss (**Table 2.8**).

Cardiac syncope This is suggested by:
- Onset within seconds
- Onset during exercise – this is a red flag for cardiac pathology
- Concurrent palpitations, chest pain, dyspnea
- Symptoms whilst sat or supine.

Ankle swelling

Ankle swelling is often due to edema (see page 119) (**Table 2.9**). Gradual onset is often due to cardiac or systemic disease, whereas acute causes include insect bite, surgery, cellulitis or deep vein thrombosis.

Arrhythmia	Character	Exacerbating factors	Relieving factors
Bradyarrhythmias	Tired, dizziness	CCB, beta-blockers, HD	Atropine, PPM, stop drugs
Ventricular ectopics	Thump or missed beat	Electrolyte disturbance, caffeine excess	Correct electrolytes, reduce caffeine
Sinus tachycardia	Fast heartbeat	Pain, exercise, anxiety, fever	Treat underlying problem
Atrial fibrillation	Fluttering in chest, dizziness, dyspnea, transient loss of consciousness	Infection, dehydration, alcohol excess, ischemia, hyperthyroidism, caffeine	Treat underlying problem, anti-arrhythmic medication, DC cardioversion, ablate focus of the arrhythmia
Atrial flutter			
AVRT/AVNRT		Stress, caffeine, alcohol	
Ventricular tachycardia		Myocardial ischemia, cardiomyopathy	

Table 2.6 Common causes of palpitations and their features. AVNRT, atrio-ventricular nodal re-entry tachycardia. AVRT, atrio-ventricular re-entry tachycardia; CCB, calcium channel blockers; HD, heart disease; PPM, permanent pacemaker

Duration of palpitation	Cause
Seconds	Ectopic beats, i.e. not serious pathology
Minutes	Atrial fibrillation/flutter, SVT or sinus tachycardia
Hours	Atrial fibrillation/flutter or SVT lasts for several hours but normally self-terminate
Days	Normally anxiety/depression.

Table 2.7 Duration of palpitations and their likely cause. SVT, supra ventricular tachycardia

Cause	Speed of onset	Recovery	Initiating events	Associated symptoms
Carotid sinus hypersensitivity	Sudden	Rapid	Turning head, shaving, tight shirt collar	Dizziness
Hypoglycemia	Gradual	Gradual	Exercise, hypoglycemics, missed meal	Sweating, tremulous
LV outflow obstruction	Sudden	Rapid	Exercise	Chest pain, palpitations
Orthostatic hypotension	Sudden	Rapid	Change in posture, anti-hypertensives	Tunnel vision, weakness
Postural orthodromic tachycardia syndrome	Sudden	Gradual	Increased heart rate on standing	CFS, IBS, JHS
Pseudo-seizure	Gradual	Rapid	Stress, trauma	psychiatric illness
Pulmonary embolus	Sudden	Gradual	Immobility, travel, trauma, surgery	Chest pain, dyspnea
Seizure	Sudden	Gradual	Fatigue, alcohol, flashing lights	Incontinence, mouth bite
Stokes–Adams attack	Sudden	Rapid	Prolonged asystole	None
Tachycardia	Sudden	Rapid	None	Chest pain, palpitations
Vasovagal syncope	Sudden	Rapid	Pain, emotion, coughing, micturition	Dizziness, weakness

Table 2.8 Features of the different causes of syncope. CFS, chronic fatigue syndrome; IBS, irritable bowel syndrome; JHS, joint hypersensitivity syndrome.

A history should confirm the location, speed of onset and any associated symptoms.

Types

Pitting edema – where a finger indentation remains for 5 seconds or more – occurs in heart failure, renal and liver disease. It worsens with gravity and improves on elevation.

Non-pitting edema occurs with lymphatic blockage (lymphedema) or hypothyroidism (myxedema), and causes a firm swelling.

Taking a history

After introducing yourself to the patient, ask their permission to take the history, choose an area of privacy and ask if you can make notes as you proceed.

Presenting complaint

Begin with open questions, such as 'what brings you to hospital today? 'Then move on to increasingly closed questions.

History of presenting complaint

This includes:
- When it started
- Duration
- Frequency
- Exacerbating or relieving factors
- Associated symptoms.

Pain should be systematically characterized (**Table 2.2**).

Past medical history

Inquire about any prior illnesses, particularly CHD risk factors:
- Hypercholesterolemia
- Diabetes
- Kidney disease
- Hypertension.

Key differentials include chronic airways disease causing breathlessness or malignancy presenting with cachexia and edema.

Cause	Pathophysiology	Onset	Associated symptoms	Symmetry
Cellulitis	Infection and inflammation	Sudden	Fever, pain and redness	Unilateral
Deep vein thrombosis	Blood clotting	Sudden	Pain, dyspnea (pulmonary embolism)	Unilateral
Heart failure	Increased venous intra-vascular hydrostatic pressure	Gradual	Dyspnea (pulmonary edema), fatigue, weight loss	Bilateral
Renal failure	Proteinuria leading to low oncotic pressure	Gradual	Dyspnea (pulmonary edema), anemic fatigue, frothy urine	Bilateral
Liver failure	Low serum albumin leading to low oncotic pressure	Gradual	Jaundice, abdominal swelling and easy bruising	Bilateral
Myxedema/hypothyroidism	Accumulation of mucin leading to non-pitting edema	Gradual	Weight gain, neck (thyroid) swelling and fatigue	Bilateral
Pregnancy	Increased hydrostatic and decreased oncotic pressure	Gradual		Bilateral
Travel	Prolonged immobility, decreased lymphatic and venous return	Sudden	None, but at risk of DVT/pulmonary embolism	Bilateral

Table 2.9 Causes of ankle edema and their features. DVT, deep vein thrombosis.

Drug history

This includes recent medications, dosage, route and frequency:
- Use full generic names
- Be clear on dosages
- Include over-the-counter and alternative medications.

Common cardiotoxins include non-steroidal anti-inflammatory drugs (NSAIDs), anabolic steroids, radiotherapy and chemotherapeutic agents.

Allergy history

Allergies may include drugs, latex, peanuts, shellfish or other substances. Specify the drug, route, nature and severity of the reaction. Side effects should also be noted.

Family medical history

Construct a family tree to document any heritable conditions (**Table 2.10**) in first-degree relatives, including MI or sudden cardiac death in those under 60 years.

> ### Guiding principle
> Smokers should always be encouraged to stop and be provided with sufficient information and support to aid cessation.

Social history

Occupation Some occupations, e.g. owning a bar, are associated with cardiovascular risk factors. It is also important to be aware of how disease or a diagnosis may limit livelihood.

Smoking Smoking is the biggest risk factor for cardiovascular disease. One 'pack year' is 20 cigarettes a day for 1 year.

Alcohol Record weekly consumption in units. Moderate alcohol consumption appears beneficial for cardiovascular health, but regular and excessive consumption leads to dilated cardiomyopathy and/or rhythm disturbance such as AF.

Caffeine Excessive caffeine consumption can lead to sinus tachycardia or ectopic beats.

Recreational drugs Amphetamines are sympathomimetic and can cause palpitations and hypertension. Cocaine can

Disorder	Inheritance	Complications
Arryhthmogenic right ventricular dysplasia	AD	SCD, arrhythmia
Amyloidosis	AD	Heart block, heart failure
Brugada's syndrome	AD	SCD, arrhythmia
Long QT	AD/R	SCD, arrhythmia
Hypertrophic cardiomyopathy	AD	SCD, arrhythmia
Dilated cardiomyopathy	AD/R	Heart failure, arrhythmia
Marfan's syndrome	AD	MVP, aortopathy
Atrial myxoma	AD	Stroke, syncope

Table 2.10 Inherited cardiac conditions. AD, autosomal dominant; AD/R, autosomal dominant/recessive; HF, heart failure; MVP, mitral valve prolapse; SCD, sudden cardiac death.

lead to coronary artery spasm, thrombosis, myocarditis and sudden death.

Functional capacity Functional capacity should be regularly documented to monitor changes and influence decisions of treatment and prognosis. Ask about mobility, what type of home they live in and if they have any help.

Exercise Atherosclerosis is associated with a sedentary lifestyle; exercise helps lower blood pressure, increase energy and decrease depression.

Guiding principle

All patients should be encouraged to exercise a minimum of 30 min of moderate exercise five times a week.

Systems review

A systems review ensures that nothing relevant is missed (**Table 2.11**).

Guiding principle

Avoid interrupting patients: the diagnosis is usually given to you in the history.

Summary

Briefly summarize the history back to the patient to check the facts have been recorded correctly. Lastly, ask the patient if they have any questions, concerns or expectations.

System	Sign/symptom	Cardiac and related causes
Respiratory	Cough	Infection, heart failure or angiotensin converting enzyme inhibitors
	Wheeze	Cardiac asthma due to heart failure
	Hemoptysis	Pulmonary embolism, pulmonary edema or mitral stenosis
	Stroke	Following aortic dissection or atrial fibrillation
Endocrine	Changes in mood, weight or energy	Thyroid disease
	Sweating, weakness and headaches	Adrenal disease
Musculoskeletal	Myalgia	Statins, unaccustomed exercise or tissue ischemia
Neurological	Dizziness	Postural hypotension
	Syncope	Cardiac diseases e.g. aortic stenosis and medications e.g. anti-hypertensive agents
	Headache	Cardiac medication, e.g. nitrates
	Stroke	Aortic dissection, atrial fibrillation
Gastrointestinal	Weight loss	Cardiac cachexia – a poor prognostic indicator
	Gastric reflux	Cardiac drugs causing chest pain
	Diarrhea	Arrhythmia due to loss of potassium
	Nausea and vomiting	Complication of MI
Genitourinary	Impotence	Underlying vascular disease
	Hematuria	Glomerulonephritis or endocarditis
	Proteinuria	Peripheral edema due to renal disease
	Frequency	Prostatic disease or diuretic use

Table 2.11 Systems review: key clinical features associated with cardiac disease.

2.2 Cardiovascular examination

Clinical examination requires a systematic routine (**Table 2.12**).

Starting the examination

To prepare:
- Wash your hands, introduce yourself and check the patient's identity
- Obtain verbal consent for 'a heart and chest examination, which will require removal of clothing from the waist upwards'
- Ensure modesty is preserved and, if appropriate, ask if the patient would like a chaperone
- Position the patient at 45°.

General inspection

Carefully survey the patient and surroundings:
- Does the patient look well, i.e. pink, talkative, smiling, not in pain or distress?
- Are there any medications or other treatments present?

Hands

Ask the patient to rest their hands on a pillow.

Finger clubbing

Digital clubbing is characterized by increased soft tissue

> **Clinical insight**
>
> The hands convey a great deal of information about a patient, for example: signs of chronic disease, circulation, occupation, hobbies, smoking, hygiene, nervousness and strength.

and vasodilation (**Figure 2.2**, **Table 2.13**) and is a sign of chronic pulmonary, cardiac, liver or gastrointestinal disease that increases circulating growth factors.

Cardiac causes include:
- Benign cardiac tumors
- Cyanotic congenital heart disease
- Infective endocarditis.

Signs of infective endocarditis

Infective endocarditis can present with finger signs (**Figure 2.3**).

System or category	Examination	Signs
General inspection	Appearance	Systemically well or unwell, underweight (cachexia), overweight or obese
	Environment	Clues suggesting disease
	Face	Central cyanosis (blue discoloration)
	Neck	Visible jugular venous pulse (fluid overload)
	Chest	Breathlessness at rest
Hands	Nails	Nail abnormalities
	Fingers	Peripheral cyanosis (bluish discoloration)
Arterial pulse	Palpation	Heart rate and rhythm
Respiration	Inspection	Respiratory rate Breathing pattern
Head and neck	Inspection	Central cyanosis (blue discoloration of the lips or tongue) Xanthelasma Jugular venous pulse
Chest	Inspection	Surgical scars, pacemakers or chest wall deformities
	Palpation	Apex beat Heaves Thrills
	Auscultation	Heart sounds Murmurs Pericardial rub Lung signs: wheeze, crepitations, dullness
Lower limb	Inspection	Xanthomata Ankle edema
	Palpation	Ankle edema Peripheral pulses
Abdomen	Inspection	Ascites
	Palpation	Ascites Abdominal aorta
	Auscultation	Renal arteries
Blood pressure		Hypertension
Fundi	Inspection	Hypertensive and diabetic retinopathy

Table 2.12 A systematic approach to cardiovascular examination.

Figure 2.2 Finger clubbing.

Stage	Description
1	Increased sponginess of the nail bed
2	Loss of the nail angle (usually < 165 degrees)
3	Increased convexity of the nail bed
4	Thickening of finger (drumstick appearance)
5	Shiny aspect and striation of finger and nail

Table 2.13 The stages of clubbing.

Figure 2.3 Signs of infective endocarditis. (a) A small splinter hemorrhage. (b) Janeway lesion.

Splinter hemorrhages are short, thin, linear discolorations in the nail that are initially red then brown and finally black within a few days. Most are due to trauma, but they can be a sign of micro-emboli from vasculitis or infective endocarditis.

Osler nodes are tender, raised, purple papules in the finger pulps, due to immune complex deposition.

Janeway lesions are non-tender, flat, purple, macules found in the palm of the hand due to septic emboli.

Palmar erythema

Reddening of the thenar and hypothenar eminences of the palm occurs with:

- Pregnancy: palmar erythema arises in 30% of pregnant women due to increased estrogen
- Polycythemia, as a manifestation of the increased number of red blood cells
- Syphilis and vasculitis, i.e. inflammation.

Peripheral cyanosis

Cyanosis is the blue discoloration associated with low oxygen. Peripheral cyanosis (**Figure 2.4**) occurs with:

- Reduced central circulation – central cyanosis (e.g. blue tongue)
- Cold
- Acute limb ischemia
- Arterial vasospasm.

Figure 2.4 Peripheral cyanosis.

Capillary refill time

Press the fingernail for 5 seconds; it should return to 'normal' within 2 seconds. A delay suggests reduced peripheral perfusion, for example:

- Cardiogenic shock
- Heart failure
- Dehydration
- Acute limb ischemia.

Arterial pulse

The arterial pulse gives information on heart rate, rhythm, cardiac output, and heart valve and vascular function.

Radial pulse

The radial pulse is felt between the radial styloid and the palmaris longus and flexor digitorum superficialis tendons.

Heart rate Palpate for 1 minute using the index and middle finger and count the beats per minute (bpm) (**Table 2.14**).

Pulse rhythm A pulse can be regularly irregular, where the period varies but has a pattern, or irregularly irregular, where there is no pattern (**Table 2.15**).

Collapsing (waterhammer) pulse Elevate the arm above the patient's head; a collapsing radial pulse of aortic regurgitation rapidly increases and collapses to feel like it is knocking against your fingertips.

Rate (bpm)	Term	Causes
< 60	Bradycardia	Sleep, hypothermia, hypothyroidism, athletic training, arrhythmia, medication
60–100	Normal	–
>100	Tachycardia	Pain, anxiety, fever, exercise, arrhythmia, shock, hyperthyroidism

Table 2.14 Causes of slow and fast heart rates.

Rhythm	Description	Causes
Regularly regular	Consistent time between each pulse	Sinus rhythm, 1st or 3rd degree heart block
Regularly irregular	Period varies but has a pattern	Sinus arrhythmia, 2nd degree heart block
Irregularly irregular	No pattern	Atrial and ventricular ectopic beats, AF, atrial flutter with variable block, MAT

Table 2.15 Causes of cardiac rhythms. AF, atrial fibrillation; MAT, multi-focal atrial tachycardia.

Delayed pulses These include:
• Radio-radial delay, which suggests aortic dissection proximal to the left subclavian artery
• Radio-femoral delay, which suggests coarctation (i.e. narrowing) of the aortic arch distal to the subclavian arteries.

Carotid pulse
Palpate the carotid pulse in the anterior cervical triangle, between the trachea and the sternocleidomastoid muscle, to assess pulse character and volume.

Pulse character Assess for changes in pulse waveform, including the slow rising, broad pulse of aortic stenosis and the collapsing, narrow pulse of aortic regurgitation (**Figure 2.5**).

Pulse volume A low volume or 'thready' pulse can reflect a reduced stroke volume felt in shock, heart failure, anxiety, and anemia or reduced vascular resistance associated with hyperthermia and hyperthyroidism.

Respiration
A normal respiratory rate is 12–20 breaths per minute. To avoid distortion, observe the rate and breathing pattern whilst still palpating the radial pulse (**Table 2.16**).

Figure 2.5 Pulse character and pulse pressure.

Head and neck
Inspect the hair, skin eyes and mouth (**Table 2.17**).

Jugular venous pulse

> ## Clinical insight
> A patient cannot be anemic and cyanotic at the same time. In fact, many cyanotic patients have compensatory polycythemia, a raised red cell count.

Moving down to the neck, examine the pulse of the internal jugular vein as an indicator of central venous pressure (CVP) (**Figure 2.6**):
- Position the patient at an angle of 45°, with their head turned to the left
- Observe the supraclavicular fossa and anterior cervical triangle on the patient's right for the characteristic double wave-form, distinct from the carotid pulse
- The JVP should be <3 cm vertically above the sternal angle. 3 cm is equivalent to 3 cm H_2O (2 mmHg).

Raised JVP The JVP is normally hidden behind the right clavicle. It is increased in:
- Biventricular/right heart failure
- Right ventricular infarction
- Fluid overload.

> ## Guiding principle
> The internal jugular vein drains directly into the right atrium, and so is a barometer of right atrial and CVP.

Sign	Definition	Causes
Bradypnea	Respiratory rate <12 breaths/min	Hypertension, hypothyroidism, decreased ICP, sedatives
Tachypnea	RR >20 breaths/min	Fever/infection, pain, anxiety, heart failure, hyperthyroidism, pulmonary embolism, pulmonary edema, pneumothorax, ILD, COPD, asthma, sympathomimetics
Dyspnea	Shortness of breath	Heart failure, asthma, COPD
Rapid shallow breathing		Pleuritic chest pain, ILD, hyperventilation
Stridor	Inspiratory wheeze	Upper airway obstruction
Kussmaul's breathing	Rapid deep sighing; 'air hunger'	Acidosis (e.g. diabetic ketoacidosis)
Excess abdominal / accessory muscle movement on inspiration		COPD, respiratory distress
Cheyne–Stokes breathing	5–30 seconds of apnea followed by increased and then decrease RR	Severe pulmonary edema and brainstem lesions
Prolonged expiratory phase		Significant airway obstruction due to asthma or COPD etc.

Table 2.16 Signs of respiratory rate and breathing pattern and their causes. RR, respiratory rate; ICP, intracranial pressure; ILD, interstitial lung disease; COPD, chronic obstructive pulmonary disease.

JVP waveform In sinus rhythm, two waves are visible: the 'a' wave before the carotid pulse and the 'v' wave after it (**Figure 2.7**). Pathologies include an absent 'a' wave due to atrial fibrillation (AF; **Table 2.18**).

Area	Sign	Indication
Hair	Brown tar stains	Smoking
Skin	Malar erythema	Mitral stenosis, systemic lupus erythematosus
	Gray cheekbones	Amiodarone, an antiarrhythmic agent
Eyes	Xanthelasma – yellow fat deposits in the skin around the eyes (see Figure 2.11)	Hypercholesteremia
	Corneal arcus – white ring of lipid deposits in the cornea	Hypercholesteremia, old age
	Subconjunctival pallor (pale under eyelids)	Anemia
Mouth	Dental caries (tooth decay)	Risk factor for bacterial endocarditis
	Central cyanosis	Deoxygenated hemoglobin >5.0 g/dL (> 50 g/L) chronic lung disease, myocardial infarction, congenital heart disease, or cardiogenic shock
	Pale mucus membranes	Anemia

Table 2.17 Signs of the hair, skin, eyes and mouth.

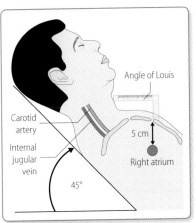

Figure 2.6 Observing the jugular venous pulse (JVP). The internal jugular vein courses from the ear lobe to between the sternal and clavicular head of sternocleidomastoid muscle at the clavicle. Note that the JVP is best observed with the patient's head turned to the left (not shown here).

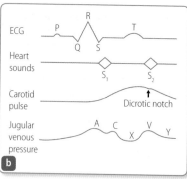

Figure 2.7 The JVP waveform (a) The waveform and its relation to the cardiac cycle. (b) The JVP and its relation to ECG, heart sounds and carotid pulse.

Wave	Descent	Meaning	Physiology	Pathology
A		RA systole.	Retrograde venous flow	Big in TS, absent in AF
C		RV contraction	TV bulges into RA	–
	X	RA diastole	TV pulled down by RV	–
V		RA diastole	Venous filling of RA	Big in TR
	Y	TV open	Fall in RA pressure	Deep in CP

Table 2.18 Waves of the JVP and pathologies that affect them. AF, atrial fibrillation; CP, constrictive pericarditis; RA, right atrium; RV, right ventricle; TS, tricuspid stenosis; TR, tricuspid regurgitation; TV, tricuspid valve.

Chest
Inspection

Inspect the shape of the anterior chest, including pectus carinatum (pigeon chest) and excavatum (hollow chest),

> ## Clinical insight
>
> Inspection involves observing not just with the eyes, but also other senses. For example, noticing the metallic clicking sound of a metallic valve replacement.

scars (**Figure 2.8**), masses, and observe its movement for regularity, symmetricality and speed.

Palpation

Apex beat The apex of the heart is the most lateral and inferior part of the heart. It transmits a pulse – the apex beat – to the chest wall, usually in the 5th intercostal space (ICS) in the mid-clavicular line (**Figure 2.9**):
- Palpate the sternal angle; the 2nd ICS is lateral to this
- Count down to the 5th ICS and across to the mid-clavicular line on the left side
- With the index finger parallel to the ribs, feel the intercostal space for the forceful pulse
- Assess for abnormalities (**Table 2.19**)

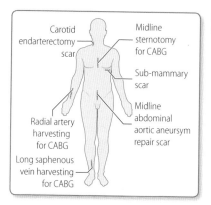

Figure 2.8 Surgical scars of cardiovascular surgery.

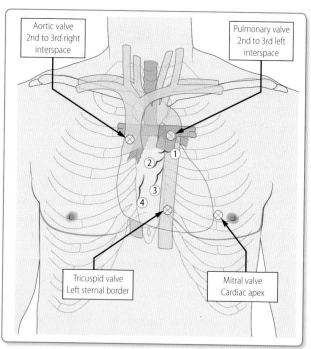

Figure 2.9 Location of the auscultation and palpation areas of the apex beat and heart valves. ① pulmonary valve; ② aortic valve; ③ bicuspid (mitral) valve; ④ tricuspid valve.

Sign	Interpretation	Cause
Displaced	LV dilation	DCM, LV aneurysm, LVSD, chest wall deformities, CLD
Tapping	Loud S1	MS
Heaving	LV pressure overload	AS, HTN, LVH
Thrusting	LV volume overload	AR, iatrogenic fluid overload
Absent	Not palpable	Normal in 50%, dextrocardia, obesity, pericardial effusion
Double beat	Forceful LA contraction	HCM

Table 2.19 Common abnormalities of the apex beat and their cause. AR, aortic regurgitation; AS, aortic stenosis; CLD, chronic lung disease; HCM, hypertrophic cardiomyopathy; HTN, hypertension; LA, left atrium; LV, left ventricle; LVH, left ventricular hypertrophy; LVSD, left ventricular systolic dysfunction; MS, mitral stenosis.

Heaves Palpate the left parasternum with the right palm for a strong cardiac impulse, which can indicate right ventricular hypertrophy (RVH) due to pulmonary hypertension or pulmonary stenosis.

Thrills Assess the four valve areas (**Figure 2.9**) with fingertips for palpable murmurs; high-frequency vibrations.

Auscultation

Heart sounds Listen with a stethoscope to the four valve areas (**Figure 2.9**), with both the diaphragm (best for high pitch, e.g. aortic and mitral regurgitation) and the bell (better for low pitch, e.g. aortic and mitral stenosis). While auscultating, palpate the carotid pulse to orientate where sounds are occurring in the cardiac cycle.

Heart sounds reflect the valves shutting: S1 and S2 are

Clinical insight

There is no direct correlation between murmur volume and the echocardiographic severity of the lesion.

Clinical insight

A 'gallop rhythm' is the sound of all four heart sounds, S1 to S4 ('le-lup-de-dup') and is typically due to decompensated chronic or acute heart failure.

normally the most obvious (**Table 2.20**). S3 and S4 are 'added heart sounds' and can represent pathology.

S2 split is when S2 consists of two separate sounds as the left ventricle typically contracts before the right ventricle: A2 when the aortic valve shuts, and P2 when the pulmonary valve does. This 'splitting' of S2 varies according to how it is affected by ventilation (**Table 2.21**).

Heart murmurs Murmurs are the sound of turbulent blood flow through heart valves, forward or backward. Forward murmurs reflect a narrowing; backward murmurs indicate valve incompetence (**Table 2.22** and **Figure 2.10**).

Pericardial rub This is a sign of pericarditis, when two layers of inflamed pericardium rub against each other, said to sound like the crunching sound of walking on fresh snow.

Lungs

After auscultating the heart, ask the patient to sit forward and examine the lung bases, using inspection, palpation, auscultation and percussion.

Sound	Phonetic	Interpretation
S1	'lup'	Shutting of mitral and tricuspid valves at the start of ventricular systole, when the ventricular pressures rise above the atria
S2	'dup'	Shutting of aortic and pulmonary valves at the end of ventricular systole, when ventricular pressure falls below that of the aorta and pulmonary artery
S3	'lup-de-dup'	In diastole, between S2 and S1. Normal in children or young adults but can indicate rapid ventricular filling in heart failure
S4	'le-lup-dup'	Always abnormal, due to a stiff ventricle, normally secondary to left ventricular hypertrophy

Table 2.20 Heart sounds.

S2 split	Pathologies	Mechanism	Split order
Normal inspiration split	None	Inspiration reduces intrathoracic pressure and increases venous return to RA, delaying P2	A2 occurs before P2
Abnormal expiration split	Electrophysiological pathology (e.g. LBBB), structural heart disease (e.g. aortic stenosis) or cardiomyopathy	Prolonged LV ejection	P2 occurs before A2
Abnormal inspiration and expiration 'fixed' split	ASD, VSD	Independent of ventilation, septal defects shunt blood from left to right circulation, down the pressure gradient, so that the RV ejection is delayed	A2 occurs before P2

Table 2.21 Splitting of S2. RA, right atrium. LBBB, left bundle branch block. ASD, atrial septal defect. VSD. Ventricular septal defect.

Stage of cycle	Murmur	Timing	Sound	Location	Radiation
Systole	AS	Ejection	Crescendo–decrescendo	2nd R ICS	Carotid
	MR	Pan	Blowing	5th L ICS	Axilla
Diastole	AR	Early	Decrescendo	2nd L ICS	Carotid
	MS	Mid	Rumbling	5th L ICS	Axilla

Table 2.22 Detection of heart murmurs. L, left, MR, mitral regurgitation, MS, mitral stenosis, R, right, AR, aortic regurgitation, AS, aortic stenosis, ICS, inter-costal space.

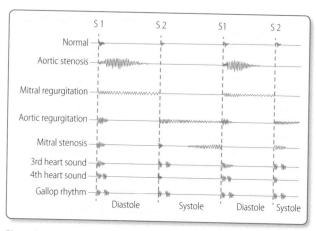

Figure 2.10 Normal and abnormal heart sounds.

Clinical insight

Physiological (flow or innocent) murmurs are typically:

- Soft
- Heard all over the precordium
- Pan-systolic
- Absent on standing (i.e. with a decrease in venous return).

Wheeze Cardiac asthma is a coarse, whistling sound heard during expiration due to obstruction of the small airways due to pulmonary edema secondary to left ventricular failure.

Crepitations These are a crackling sound like Velcro, heard at the posterior bases of the lungs. It is a sign of pulmonary edema, often secondary to left ventricular failure. The sound is most pronounced in inspiration as small airways and alveoli 'pop' open.

Stony dullness Stony dullness – a lack of resonance on percussion – in the lung bases suggests pleural effusion, a sign of heart failure that also presents with reduced chest expansion and quiet breath sounds.

Lower limb

Inspection

Inspect the skin and large extensor tendons for yellow xanthomata (**Figure 2.11**), nodular cholesterol-rich deposits that are a sign of hypercholesterolemia.

Ankle edema Excess interstitial fluid, i.e. edema, is caused by chronic disease that affects blood hydrostatic or oncotic pressure or localized disease affecting fluid build-up and return (**Table 2.9**). Heart failure is a cause of bilateral pitting edema, or sacral edema in bed-bound patients, due to fluid retention from decreased hydrostatic pressure.

Ulcers Inspect the lower limb for ulcers (**Figure 2.12**); a sign of peripheral vascular disease (PVD). Arterial PVD is commonly due to diabetes, hypertension and smoking.

> ## Guiding principle
>
> Heart failure is effectively a pump failure that leads to back-pressure and fluid leakage:
> - Left-sided failure – leakage in pulmonary circulation causes pulmonary edema
> - Right-sided failure – leakage into interstitial space causing peripheral edema (ankle and sacral edema)
> - As right-sided failure worsens, leakage can occur into the abdomen causing ascites.

Figure 2.11 Xanthomata lipid deposits. Xanthelasma are small xanthoma around eyelids.

Figure 2.12 Arterial ulcers are usually deep, regular, painful, and have minimal exudate.

Palpation

Pulses Palpate the four pulses in each lower limb (**Figure 2.13**):
- Femoral artery
- Popliteal artery
- Posterior tibial
- Dorsalis pedis.

Pulse absence suggests PVD due to atherosclerosis, typically with peripheral pulses lost first.

Calf tenderness Gently squeeze both calves to assess for pain due to deep vein thrombosis (DVT), which will also present with edema, and possibly warmth, pain and erythema.

Clinical insight

The presence of atherosclerosis in the lower limb (peripheral vascular disease) reflects the likely presence of atherosclerosis in the carotid and coronary arteries; i.e. PVD indicates the risk of coexisting cerebrovascular and cardiovascular disease.

Abdomen

Examine the abdomen for fluid, and aortic or renal artery disease.

Inspection A distended abdomen may indicate ascites due to advanced right or biventricular failure, as back-pressure in portal veins leads to fluid leak, though the vast majority is associated with liver cirrhosis or GI malignancy.

Palpation Palpate for the presence of a midline, central and possibly tender, pulsatile mass – a sign of abdominal aortic aneurysm (AAA).

Auscultation Listen for a renal artery bruit (turbulent blood flow) anteriorly at positions 9 and 3 o'clock, 5 cm from the umbilicus, otherwise posteriorly paraspinal at level of L2. This is a sign of renal artery stenosis, a cause of secondary hypertension and sudden pulmonary edema.

Blood pressure

Blood pressure is an estimate of the force that blood is exerting against the walls of the large arteries. It used to gauge disease severity in cases of blood loss and in aortic valve diseases, and to diagnose, monitor and manage hypertension.

Figure 2.13 Pulses of the lower limb: the femoral, popliteal, posterior and anterior tibial arteries. (a) (1) femoral nerve, (2) femoral artery and vein, (3) sartorius, (4) adductor longus, (X) pubic tubercle. (b) (1) Common fibular nerve, (2) tibial nerve, (3) popliteal vein, (4) popliteal artery. (c) (1) Posterior tibial tendon, (2) flexor digitorum longus, (3) flexor hallucis longus, (4) posterior tibial artery, (5) tibial nerve, (6) flexor retinaculum. (d) (1) Anterior tibial artery, (2) anterior tibial tendon, (3) inferior extensor retinaculum, (4) medial branch of deep fibular nerve, (5) dorsalis pedis artery, (6) arcuate artery, (7) extensor hallucis longus tendon.

Whether it is measured with an automated monitor or a sphygmomanometer and a stethoscope, the positioning of the patient and the cuff is the same:

- Ask the patient to remain still and rest their arm on a desk or similar

- Place the cuff around the patient's upper arm, approximately at heart-height
- Place the diaphragm over the brachial artery

If the measurement is being taken with a sphygmomanometer:

- Inflate the cuff until the radial pulse is obliterated
- Listen as the cuff is steadily deflated
- Record the pressure at which Korotkoff sounds of turbulent flow are heard: this is the highest, systolic pressure (SBP)
- Record the pressure at which they disappear: this is the lowest, diastolic pressure (DBP).

Pulse pressure

$$Pulse\ pressure = SBP - DBP$$

Pulse pressure (Figure 2.6) is normally 40–80 mmHg.

Narrow pulse pressure Pressures <40 mmHg occur if there is an increase in LV afterload (e.g. aortic stenosis, cardiac tamponade and cardiogenic shock) or a reduction in LV contractility (e.g. heart failure) causing a reduction in volume or speed of ejection of blood from the LV during systole.

Broad pulse pressure Pressures > 80 mmHg occur when there is a reduction in LV afterload (e.g. aortic regurgitation, pregnancy, fever, thyroxicosis, AV malformation and Paget's disease) causing a rapid dispersion of blood from the LV during systole.

Mean arterial pressure (MAP)

$$MAP = DBP + (1/3\ pulse\ pressure)$$

MAP is the average blood pressure throughout the cardiac cycle and represents the perfusion pressure supplying organs. It is normally 70–110 mmHg; <70 mmHg leads to tissue ischemia, infarction and eventually necrosis.

Blood pressure symmetry

A difference of systolic blood pressure between arms of more than 20 mmHg is usually a sign of aortic dissection.

Fundi

Fundoscopy is performed in a darkened room with an ophthalmoscope to view the retinae.

Diabetic retinopathy

This can present with edema (yellow exudate), retinal and vitreous hemorrhages and new vessels (**Table 2.23**, **Figure 2.14**).

Hypertensive retinopathy

Fundoscopy can reveal diffuse or focal vessel narrowing, microaneurysms, macroaneurysms, cotton wool spots, exudates and disc swelling (**Figure 2.15**, **Table 2.24**).

> ### Clinical insight
>
> The presence of retinal microvascular disease likely reflects microvascular disease in other organs.

Stage	Features
Early diabetic retinopathy	Microaneurysms, dot hemorrhages, blot hemorrhages, yellow exudate, cotton wool spots
Preproliferative retinopathy	More severe
Proliferative diabetic retinopathy	New vessels
Diabetic maculopathy	Macular disease: exudate, hemorrhage, edema

Table 2.23 Stages of diabetic retinopathy.

Figure 2.14 Proliferative diabetic retinopathy, with evidence of new vessel formation.

Figure 2.15 Severe, grade 4 hypertensive retinopathy: silver wiring ①; arteriovenous (AV) nipping ②; cotton wool spots ③; flame hemorrhages ④; hard exudate ⑤; optic disc edema ⑥.

Grade	Sign	Pathophysiology
I	Silver/copper wiring	Visible atherosclerosis; tortuous and shiny arterioles
II	Arteriovenous nipping	Venous constriction
III	Cotton-wool spots and flame hemorrhages	Retinal infarcts and bleeds
IV	Papilledema	Compression of the central retinal vein swells the optic disk

Table 2.24 Grading of signs of hypertensive retinopathy.

2.3 Investigations

Investigations support or refute the working diagnoses, determine disease severity and inform a management plan.

Blood tests

Routine tests include:
- Complete blood count (CBC) to assess for anemia, inflammation and infection
- Urea and electrolytes (U&E) to assess renal function
- Liver function tests (LFT)
- Clotting screen to assess for coagulopathies.

Cardiac biomarkers

Cardiac biomarkers are molecules released into the blood when myocardial cells are damaged (**Figure 2.16**, **Table 2.25**). They are measured as soon as possible after a suspected cardiac event, e.g. chest pain and suspected MI; dyspnea and suspected heart failure, to obtain a baseline level.

> ### Clinical insight
>
> Natriuretic peptides are raised in hypertension and also:
> - Renal failure
> - Pulmonary embolus
> - Myocardial infarction
> - Sepsis
> - Extreme exercise.

Lipid profiles

Inherited or acquired raised serum lipids are a risk factor for vascular disease. Concentrations are measured in a venous blood sample after overnight fasting.

Low-density lipoprotein (LDL) Often called 'bad cholesterol' in conversations with patients, this carries cholesterol from the liver to the peripheries (see page 80). It is associated with cholesterol deposition in arteries to form atheroma.
- Normally <2.5 mmol/L (<100 mg/dL)

Figure 2.16 Cardiac biomarkers.

Biomarker	Definition	Cardiac subtypes	Released	Measure 2nd level	Comment
Troponin	3-unit protein involved in muscle contraction	I and T	Myocardial damage	3-6 h after height of pain	
Creatine kinase	Enzyme in high–energy cells; catalyzes ATP to ADP	CK-MB	Myocardial damage	72 h after height pain	Doubling suggests MI. CK-MB is sensitive but not specific for MI
Myoglobin	Muscular form of hemoglobin (Fe- based porphyrin ring that binds O_2)		Myocardial damage	2 h	Sensitive but not specific for MI
Natriuretic peptides	Small proteins that cause sodium and water excretion	BNP and precursor NTpro-BNP	Myocardial stretch		Support a diagnosis of heart failure

Table 2.25 Cardiac biomarkers. ATP, adenosine triphosphate; ADP, adenosine diphosphate; MI, myocardial infarction; BNP, NTpro-BNP, N-terminal pro-brain naturetic peptide.

- Elevated in pregnancy, corticosteroid use, hypothyroidism and cholestatic liver disease.

High-density lipoprotein (HDL) Often called 'good cholesterol' in discussion with patients, this is the major carrier from the peripheries to the liver, and reduces cholesterol deposits in arteries. High levels are associated with a reduced risk of vascular disease.
- Normally >1.5 mmol/L (<60 mg/dL)
- Increased by exercise and modest alcohol consumption.

Triglycerides (TGs) These are esters of glycerol and three fatty acids that transfer fatty acids and glucose between fat tissue and the liver. High levels increase the risk of vascular disease.
- Normally <1.5 mmol/L (<60 mg/dL)
- Increased in diabetes, renal failure, obesity and corticosteroids.

Total cholesterol (TC) This includes LDL, HDL, VDL (variable density lipoproteins, estimated) and is normally <5 mmol/L (<200 mg/dL).

Electrocardiography (ECG)

Electrocardiography (ECG) uses electrodes placed on the chest and limbs to measure the amount and direction of the heart's electrical activity.

> **Clinical insight**
>
> Indications for ECG include chest pain, shortness of breath, palpitations, syncope, heart murmur, hypo/hypertension and an irregular pulse.

Leads

A 'lead' is the term for both the physical electrode, and the abstract positional 'view of the electrical heart' that one or more leads represents. An ECG in clinical non-acute situations is recorded using 12 leads. A 3-lead ECG is used for monitoring, whereas defibrillator paddles can also function as leads to record an ECG in acute situations.

The 12-lead ECG

A 12-lead ECG (**Figure 2.17**) is used to diagnose arrhythmias, electrolyte disturbances, myocardial disease, focal ischemia and drug toxicity. The 12-lead signals are from six chest leads and six virtual leads created from four limb leads. Results should be interpreted in a systematic way (**Table 2.26**).

Chest leads

V1–V6 view the heart in the horizontal plane from front to back. They are unipolar; they record the difference in voltage between their location on the chest, and zero.

Limb leads

The four limb leads view the electrical signal of the heart in the vertical plane (i.e. head to toe) and are colour coded:

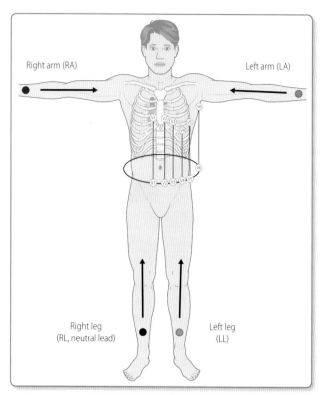

Figure 2.17 The 12-lead ECG.

- Left arm (LA) – orange
- Right arm (RA) – red
- Left leg (LL) – green
- Right leg (RL) – neutral/black

Virtual leads

Limb leads are used to create the six virtual leads; virtual perspectives of the heart's electrical activity calculated from combinations of lead measurements (**Table 2.27**).

Step	Observe
1	Patient's name, date of birth, hospital number
2	Time and date of ECG
3	Speed and voltage of ECG
4	Cardiac axis – normal or deviated?
5	Heart rate (beats/minute)
6	Heart rhythm – in normal sinoatrial rhythm, each QRS complex is preceded by a P wave
7	PQRST: examine P wave, PR interval, QRS complex, ST segment, Q waves, QT interval and T wave in each lead

Table 2.26 Interpreting a 12-lead electrocardiogram (ECG).

Unipolar leads Unipolar limb leads aVF, aVR and aVL record the electrical signal from one position, a limb, towards the center of all three leads (**Figure 2.18**), looking at the heart in an axial plane.

Bipolar leads Leads I, II and III record the electrical potential difference between 2 leads and represent a view from the positive limb lead toward the negative.

> **Clinical insight**
>
> ECG machines should be set to record at:
> - A speed of 25 mm/s: a large square (5 mm) represents 0.2 s and a small square (1 mm) is 0.04 s
> - A voltage of 0.1 mv/mm, so that 1 large square (5 mm) is 1 mv.

The ECG shape
Electricity moving towards a lead causes an upward voltage deflection; and vice versa. The more directly it is moving towards the lead, the stronger the upward deflection. Most of the electrical impulse occurs during ventricular contraction – the QRS complex (**Figure 2.19**).

Cardiac axis
As the ECG deflection represents the amount and direction of the heart's electrical activity, the cardiac axis can be

Polarity	Lead	How it is calculated	View
Unipolar	(aVF) augmented vector lead of the foot	LF − 0	From LF
	(aVR) augmented vector lead of the right arm	RA − 0	From RA
	(aVL) augmented vector lead of the left arm	LA − 0	From LA
Bipolar	I	aVR − aVL	from LA towards RA
	II	aVR − aVF	From LL towards RA
	III	aVL − aVF	from LL towards LA

Table 2.27 Virtual ECG leads.

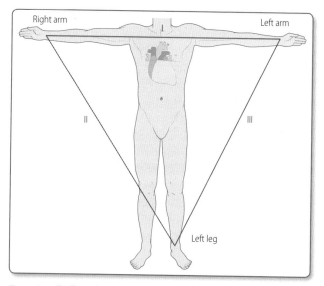

Figure 2.18 Eindhoven's triangle – the right arm, left arm, neutral and left foot give three unipolar leads aVR, aVL and aVF, creating a triangle; the bipolar leads I, II and III are the potential difference measured between each.

Figure 2.19 Waveforms and intervals of the ECG.

measured (**Figure 2.20**). It is normally −30 to +90° (11 o'clock to 5 o'clock) but can be deviated by disease (**Table 2.28**).

Analysis of the ECG

An ECG trace is analyzed for heart rate, rhythm and the shape, size and duration of characteristic deflections from the baseline, i.e. waves. Waves and the intervals between them give information about different aspects of heart function.

Heart rate The heart rate is best judged on the rhythm strip; the long lead II reading at the bottom. The rate in beats per minute (bpm) is the number of large squares between each QRS complex (the R–R interval) divided by 300.

Rhythm In sinus rhythm, P waves (atrial depolarization) are followed by QRS complexes (ventricular depolarization) with a regular PR interval between them. Absence of this interval suggests an atrial arrhythmia, causing a tachycardia; or AV node disease, causing a bradycardia (**Table 2.30**).

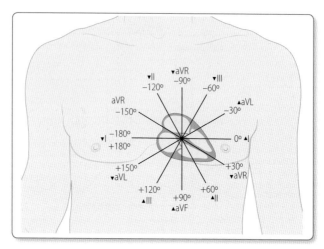

Figure 2.20 The cardiac axis.

Deviation	Examples
Right axis (+90 to +180°)	Can be normal, especially in tall, thin individuals Right bundle branch block (RBBB) Right ventricular hypertrophy (RVH) Pulmonary embolism (PE) Cor pulmonale
Left axis (–30 to –90°)	Left bundle branch block (LBBB) Left ventricular hypertrophy (LVH) Cardiac pacemaker Left anterior hemiblock

Table 2.28 Cardiac axis deviation.

BP and ECG monitoring

Hypertension and pathology affecting the ECG can be sporadic and change over time. It is therefore often necessary to monitor BP and ECG (**Table 2.29**) over periods of time for diagnosis, to gauge disease severity or measure outcomes.

Ankle–brachial pressure index This is the ratio of the systolic BP in the arms (brachial artery) to the ankle (posterior tibial artery). A negative ABPI indicates peripheral vascular disease causing a relative decrease in leg blood pressure.

> ## Guiding principle
> Atrial repolarization is hidden by the much larger ventricular depolarization (QRS complex).

> ## Clinical insight
> Enlarged Q waves represent a myocardial window of electrically inert myocardium ('dead wall') due to MI, so that the electrical signal from the opposite active heart wall is detected.

Ambulatory blood pressure monitor (ABPM) A portable sphygmomanometer measures BP at regular intervals, e.g. every 20 min, over a 24-hour period to diagnose hypertension and assess treatment.

24 hour, 48 hour, 7-day ECG, and implantable loop recorder A 3-lead ECG recorder (Holter monitor) is worn for 1–7 days; a matchbox-sized implantable loop recorder (ILR) can be used for up to 3 years.

Tilt table test This investigates autonomic dysfunction with postural changes, e.g. postural hypotension or postural orthostatic tachycardia. A patient is laid on a platform with ECG and BP monitoring as their posture is manipulated.

Exercise testing

Exercise tests are used to provoke symptoms and assess function.

6-minute walk test (6MWT) This is used to assess heart failure and pre-operative fitness. It is the distance a patient can walk on a hard, flat surface; < 500 m is abnormal.

Exercise tolerance test (ETT) In ETT, also known as the cardiac stress test, a patient exercises on a treadmill or exercise bike whilst BP and ECG data is recorded, before, during, and after

Element	Definition	Morphology	Amplitude	Duration	Pathologies
P wave	Atrial depolarization	Upward deflection before QRS	<0.2 mv (2 small squares)	<0.12 s (3 small squares)	P mitrale: bifid wave due to LA enlargement P pulmonale: tall, peaked wave due to RA enlargement
PR interval	Conduction through AVN and HPB	Region from start of the P wave and start of QRS	No deflection	0.12–0.20s (3–5 small squares)	<0.12 s = ventricular pre-excitation >0.20 s = AV block Depressed: pericarditis
Q waves	Interventricular septum depolarization (left to right)	Any negative deflection before R wave	<0.2 mV (2 small squares)	<0.04 s (1 small square)	>0.2 mV or >0.04 s = inert myocardium from MI
QRS complex	Ventricular depolarization	Region from Q to the end of S	2.5–3 mv	<0.12 s (3 small squares	Axis deviation in LVH, RVH >0.12 s seen in BBB, paced ventricular rhythm, ventricular arrhythmia or ectopic beats
ST segment	Time between ventricular depolarization and repolarization	Region between S and T waves	No deflection	0.08–0.12 s (2–3 small squares)	ST depression = ischemia ST elevation = infarction, pericarditis or LBBB

Table 2.29 *Continued...*

Element	Definition	Morphology	Amplitude	Duration	Pathologies
T wave	Ventricular repolarization	Positive deflections after each QRS complex Inverted in AVR, V1 and V2 and any lead with negative QRS	<5 mm in limb leads, <15 mm in precordial leads	<0.2 s (5 small squares).	Inverted T waves in other leads suggest ischemia or structural heart disease Tall and narrow T waves are seen in hyperkalemia Tall asymmetrical T waves are seen in STEMI in STEMI
QT interval	Ventricular depolarization and repolarization	Start of QRS to end of T wave QT corrected (QTc) for heart rate = QT/square root of the RR interval (in seconds)	No deflection	QTc <0.40 s (10 small squares) in women and <0.45 s (11 small squares) in men	Prolonged QT is rarely genetic and commonly drug-induced. risk of arrhythmias
U wave	Abnormal	Bifid small positive deflection immediately after T wave			Hypokalemia
J wave	Abnormal	Positive wave just after QRS			Hypothermia

Table 2.29 ECG elements. LA, left atrium; RA, right atrium; AVN, atrioventricular node; HPB, His-Purkinje bundle; LVH, eft ventricular hypertrophy; RVH, right ventricular hypertrophy.

Pathology	Disease	Pathophysiology	ECG signs
Atrial arrhythmias	Atrial fibrillation	No organized electrical activity	No discernible P wave
	Atrial flutter	Re-entrant circuit in the atria	Saw-tooth baseline, comprising flutter (F) waves before each QRS
Heart (AV) block	First degree	Delay in AV conduction	P wave before each QRS but the PR interval is prolonged
	2nd degree	Some P waves not conducted by the AV node	Mobitz type I: PR interval progressively prolonged until a P wave is 'dropped' Mobitz type II: 2–3 P waves before each QRS
	Third degree (complete)	No conduction across the AV node; depolarization originates in ventricles	Bradycardia with no relationship between atrial (P wave) and ventricular (QRS) electrical activity

Table 2.30 Atrial arrhythmias and heart block on ECG. AV, atrioventricular.

exercise to a set target, such as maximal heart rate (max heart rate = 220 – age in years). It is used to:
- Diagnose CHD (when CT calcium scoring is not available) – a diagnosis is confirmed by observing horizontal ST depression in more than one lead
- Monitor rehabilitation after MI
- Detect arrhythmias

Cardiopulmonary exercise testing (CPET) This is the assessment of cardiorespiratory fitness, and is used to assess the need for transplant in heart failure and for pre-operative risk assessment. The patient exercises while connected to an ECG, BP and breathing apparatus which records gas exchange and the exercise taken in terms of wattage. The maximal uptake of oxygen per kg of body mass per minute at peak exertion (Vo_2) – is recorded (**Table 2.31**).

Imaging

Cardiac imaging is used to diagnose CHD, valve disease and to assess ventricular function. CHD is assessed with:
- An anatomical study, such as a coronary angiography, to locate the atherosclerotic lesion
- A functional study, such as stress echocardiography, to demonstrate the lesion's physiological *consequences*.

Chest radiography

Chest radiography is used to visualize changes in heart size and shape, thoracic vessels and lung fields, including signs of:
- Heart failure – cardiomegaly, pleural effusion, pulmonary edema, pulmonary hypertension, ventricular hypertrophy
- Constrictive pericarditis – calcification of the pericardium
- Aortic dissection – widened mediastinum
- Pleural effusions – blunting of the costophrenic angles
- Remnants of interventions e.g. sternal wires, artificial valves, LV assist devices and pacemakers.

Ultrasound

Ultrasound uses high frequency sound waves (>20 mHz) to visualize tissues and organs. The waves pass

Clinical insight

If there is cardiomegaly (i.e. a cardiothoracic ratio > 50% on a PA view) look for other signs of heart failure

Vo_2 (mL/kg/min)	Patient groups
>70	Elite athletes
>50	Healthy active individuals
>30	Healthy sedentary individuals
<20	Pre-transplant heart failure

Table 2.31 Cardiopulmonary exercise testing: typical Vo_2 values for different patient groups.

through less-dense structures such as blood and air, but are reflected by denser structures such as muscle and bone. Reflections are detected by the transducer and transformed into a digital image. It is cheap, quick and involves no radiation.

Carotid Doppler ultrasound This uses the Doppler effect of sound waves to visualize blood movement; the frequency is higher as it travels towards the transducer and lower as it moves away. It is used to locate and quantify the degree of artery narrowing due to atherosclerosis, particularly in the carotid arteries following a stroke or before a coronary artery bypass graft (CABG).

Abdominal ultrasound This is the first choice to assess for the presence, location and size of an AAA, but does not visualize the entire abdominal aorta.

Venous duplex ultrasound This is used to visualize venous anatomy and blood flow, for example, in diagnosing DVT, typically in patients with a unilateral painful and swollen leg.

Echocardiography

Echocardiography uses ultrasound to assess the structure and function of the heart, particularly heart muscle and valves. Indications include breathlessness, heart murmur and syncope.

Transthoracic echocardiography Transthoracic echocardiography (TTE) uses an ultrasound probe on the thoracic wall.

Motion (M) mode Pulses are emitted in quick succession in a single plane, producing a one dimensional image, a single, highly focused 'cut' through the heart, with time on the X axis and the depth from the probe on the Y. It can show rapid and small movements well, and is best for fine measurements, such as left ventricular wall thickness.

Brightness (B) mode This is the most familiar echo mode, with width displayed on the X-axis and depth on the Y-axis. The fan-shaped beam projects across the heart, producing a cross-sectional tomograph from 4 view points (**Figure 2.21**). It is used to assess:

Figure 2.21 Echocardiography 'windows'. (a) parasternal next to the left parasternal border (b) apical at the LV apex (c) subcostal from under the diaphragm (d) suprasternal from the neck.

- Valve structure and function
- Ventricular function
- Chamber size
- Masses or structural heart disease
- Pericardial disease.

Doppler echocardiography Doppler echocardiography is used to estimate blood velocity and quantify the severity of stenotic and regurgitant valvular disease (**Figure 2.22**).

3D echocardiography This is used to visualize structural heart and valve disease (**Figure 2.23**). Tissue resolution is limited compared to CT or MRI.

Trans-esophageal echocardiography An ultrasound probe is inserted into the esophagus to image posterior heart structures,

Figure 2.22
Echocardiogram
demonstrating Doppler
shift with color flow
mapping.

Figure 2.23 3D echocardiogram of the left ventricle.

including the aortic arch, mitral valve and left atrium. It is useful to visualize aortic dissection, mitral valve endocarditis and left atrial thrombus.

Stress echocardiography This is a functional investigation to induce and localize CHD, by combining echocardiography and a cardiac stressor such as exercise or a sympathomimetic drug (e.g. adenosine). It can visualize areas of the ventricle that fail to contract; a regional wall motion abnormality (RWMA) due to inadequate perfusion.

Nuclear medicine

Nuclear medicine uses intravenous radioactive contrast to visualize its uptake by tissues with a radiosensitive camera. It is used in patients with CHD, where exercise testing is contraindicated, to compare blood flow before and after administration of a sympathomimetic drug (e.g. adenosine) (**Figure 2.24**).

Computed tomography

A computer tomography (CT) scan uses ionizing X-ray radiation, reflected by tissues to varying degrees, to take tomographic (i.e. sectional) pictures of the heart and vessels. Axial sections are

Figure 2.24 Cardiac nuclear medicine: a myocardial perfusion scan of a left ventricle (LV) showing a perfusion deficit in the anterior and septal LV walls not present at rest. This indicates reversible ischemia from proximal LAD artery occlusion. ① anterior wall; ② posterior wall; ③ septal wall; ④ lateral wall.

combined to create a 3D image. CT is used to diagnose CHD, and to visualize aberrant vessels and cardiac masses such as tumors.

Coronary artery calcium score As atherosclerotic lesions calcify as they age, a low-dose CT scan is used to quantify calcification in coronary arterial walls in patients with a low likelihood of CHD (<30%):

- Low (0 Agatston units) suggests there is no CHD
- Moderate (1–400) indicates further imaging (CT angiography)
- High (>400) indicates invasive angiography.

> **Clinical insight**
>
> Calcium in arteries nearly always indicates atherosclerosis but gives no indication of plaque stability and therefore the risk of an acute coronary event.

Computed tomography coronary angiography (CTCA) This uses intravenous iodine contrast to visualize the coronary arteries. It is used to assess patients with a moderate likelihood of CHD (30–60%), and those post-CABG. It has a higher tissue resolution than CT calcium score or invasive angiography, and can visualize soft, unstable plaques.

Magnetic resonance imaging

Magnetic resonance imaging (MRI) uses a magnetic field at a specific resonance frequency to excite hydrogen atoms in the body. The resulting radio frequency signal emitted by the atoms is detected and converted into a 2D image and combined 3D image (**Figure 2.25**). Cardiac MRI (cMR) is used to assess:

- Cardiac volumes
- Right ventricular disease
- Congenital heart disease
- Post MI scar tissue (with IV contrast)
- Coronary perfusion in CHD (with IV contrast).

Cardiac catheterization

Catheterization uses X-ray imaging and a catheter that injects contrast and senses blood pressures. It is used to investigate CHD, valve diseases, and pulmonary hypertension.

Figure 2.25 Cardiac magnetic resonance scan. (1) left ventricle; (2) aortic value; (3) aorta; (4) pulmonary artery; (5) lung; (6) liver.

Catheter access The Seldinger technique of catheterization involves:

- A guide wire is passed into the right radial or femoral artery
- A sheath is placed over the wire
- The short wire is replaced with a long one, which is pushed under X-ray guidance to the coronary area of stenosis and then exchanged for a catheter
- Radio-opaque iodine-based dye is injected through the catheter to visualize the vessels.

> **Clinical insight**
>
> cMR is invaluable in patients presenting with chest pain, ischemic ECG changes, and significantly raised troponin but a normal angiogram, as it can visualize other causes such as acute cardiomyopathies.

Left heart catheterization (LHC) A LHC study includes coronary angiography, aortography and LV ventriculography, performed to investigate CHD and aortic valve disease.

Coronary angiography This uses contrast to visualize the patency and blood flow of the coronary arteries. It is normally performed in patients with a high likelihood of CHD (>60%), within <48 hours of a diagnosis of NSTEMI or within 120 minutes of presentation of a STEMI.

Aortography A pigtail catheter is used to inject contrast in multiple directions and assess the aortic valve. Reflux of contrast from the aortic root into the LV, for example, indicates aortic regurgitation.

Ventriculography A pigtail catheter is inserted into the LV and high-pressure contrast injection visualizes the shape and regional contraction of the LV. It is used to localize LV myocardial death and assess mitral regurgitation.

If left ventricular end-diastolic pressure (LVEDP) is >30 mmHg, it indicates impaired relaxation of the LV, usually due to CHD or hypertension. After ventriculography, the catheter is pulled back across the aortic valve to detect any change in pressure due to aortic stenosis.

Right heart catheterization (RHC) A RHC study measures pressures in the RA, RV, pulmonary artery and pulmonary capillary bed. It is performed to assess heart transplant recipients, suspected pulmonary hypertension and valve disease.

Pulmonary artery and capillary wedge pressure The pulmonary capillary wedge pressure (PCWP) is an estimate of the pressure in the LA, with pressures of the RA, RV and pulmonary artery measured en route. The catheter is 'wedged' in a segmental or subsegmental branch of the right or left pulmonary arteries.

PCWP, due to the high compliance of the pulmonary circulation, reflects the LA and therefore the LV filling pressure. A low PCWP (<5 mmHg) suggests the patient is fluid-depleted, and a high (>15 mmHg) that the patient is fluid overloaded.

2.4 Cardiovascular risk assessment

Cardiovascular risk assessment is the calculation of a patient's risk of CHD by the presence, absence or severity of key risk factors determined in the history, examination and investigations. Tools for risk assessment include online calculators and charts constructed from large-scale population studies.

Most calculators report a person's 10-year risk of an event; in most people a risk of 20% or over is considered high risk.

Uses

Formal risk assessment is a very useful tool in the primary prevention of CHD:

- In combination with the clinical context risk is used to guide treatment decisions
- It is proven to increase adherence to treatment and engage the patient in taking an often asymptomatic disease seriously.

In particular, scores are used to judge when to use antihypertensive and lipid-lowering medication.

Risk factors

Risk calculators and charts usually take into account the key risk factors for CHD, for example:

- Age
- Gender
- Smoking
- Diabetes mellitus or a measured blood glucose
- History of angina or MI in a first-degree relative
- Body mass index (BMI) in kg/m^2
- Systolic blood pressure
- Total and HDL cholesterol
- Ethnicity
- Presence of AF.

These values are entered into the calculator, and it gives the 10-year risk of a CHD event.

Assessment tools

Risk calculators include the American College of Cardiology (ACC)/American Heart Association's (AHA) ASCVD, the Joint

British Societies for the Prevention of cardiovascular disease's JBS3 and the National Heart, Lung and Blood Institute's CVRISK. Problems with calculators include:

- Risk overestimation in low-risk groups
- Underestimation in high-risk groups
- Inconsistencies between calculators.

The inconsistencies can result in different treatment decisions, particularly if risk assessment is being used to determine therapy. This also has economic and public health implications, and can lead to over-diagnosis and associated unnecessary anxiety and side effects from treatments.

When not to use risk assessment tools

Risk calculators and charts are only of use in patients who do not have pre-existing cardiovascular disease, i.e. for primary and not secondary prevention, and who do not have a genetic predisposition, such as familial hyperlipidemia.

2.5 Conservative management

CHD is mostly a chronic result of lifestyle and diet factors. Conservative measures aim to reduce risk factors as a means of primary prevention, and also decrease disease progression or recurrence in established disease.

Smoking cessation

Smokers are five times more likely to suffer from vascular disease than non-smokers; it is the leading preventable cause of CHD and PVD. Health professionals should regularly:

- Convey the risks
- Encourage smokers to quit
- Sign-post treatment options (e.g. nicotine replacement therapy in gum, patches or electronic cigarettes or hypnotherapy) and support services.

Exercise

Regular exercise helps to reduce many risk factors, including obesity, blood pressure and LDL cholesterol, and improves mood, cardio-respiratory fitness, HDL cholesterol and insulin sensitivity. It can reduce the risk of vascular disease by up to 50%.

> ### Clinical insight
>
> Obesity is an independent risk factor for CHD, hypertension, hyperlipidemia, and diabetes. Those with central obesity have twice the risk of MI.

All health professionals should regularly highlight the profound health benefits of exercise, with a target of 30-60 minutes of sufficient intensity to cause shortness of breath, 3–5 times a week.

Exercise can also help reverse muscle wasting, and reduce angina, claudication and dyspnea.

Alcohol

Alcohol guidelines in the UK advise daily maxima of 2–3 units for women and 3–4 units for men, as well as

> ### Clinical insight
>
> 1 unit of alcohol = 250 mL beer /cider or 125 mL wine or 25 mL spirit.

several alcohol-free days a week. More than this is considered 'harmful drinking' and can lead to alcohol dependence and its associated increased risks of, for example, heart failure, alcoholic liver disease and some cancers. A small amount of alcohol is known to reduce the risk of cardiovascular disease.

Health professionals should always assess alcohol intake and if patients drink to excess, advise them of:

- Associated risks
- A reduction in consumption
- Possible treatments, including medications, detoxification regimes, hospital admission, counseling and Alcoholics Anonymous.

Diet

A healthy, balanced and 'Mediterranean' diet rich in fruit, vegetables, grains, nuts, fish and unsaturated fats and low in red meat, sodium and saturated fat (**Figure 2.26** and Table 9.2) helps improve blood pressure and lipid profile, and reduces cardiovascular risk by up to 30%.

Patients can be referred to dieticians who can advise on the practicalities of health eating.

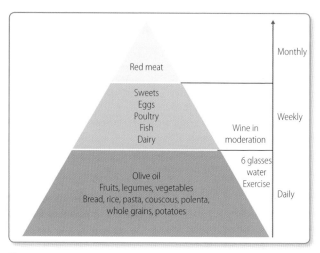

Figure 2.26 Healthy eating pyramid of a Mediterranean diet.

2.6 Medication

Patients must be made aware of:
- Why a drug is being initiated
- Possible side effects
- Monitoring requirements

Many cardiac medications require monitoring to maintain therapeutic levels and avoid harm. Warfarin is a notable example.

Lipid-lowering drugs

Hypercholesterolemia is a total cholesterol >5 mmol/L (>200 mg/dL) or LDL cholesterol >3 mmol/L (>115 mg/dL). Medication is indicated If there is no response to conservative measures, or after a diagnosis of CHD or MI. Statins are the first-line agents used to lower LDL cholesterol (**Table 2.32**). Other lipid-lowering drugs, such as fibrates and

Clinical insight

Drug selection can be daunting; consult a pharmacist, national guidelines, hospital formulary or a senior colleague before prescribing an unfamiliar medication.

Drug group	Mode of action	Effect on cholesterol	Examples	Common side effects
Statins	Inhibit HMG CoA reductase	Reduce LDL	Simvastatin Atorvastatin	Muscle aches Hepatic impairment
Fibrates	Activate PPAR receptors	Reduce LDL and TG	Bezafibrate Gemfibrozil	Indigestion Rash
Brush border lipase inhibitors	Inhibit gut absorption of lipid	Reduce LDL	Ezetimibe	Diarrhea Headache
Bile acid sequestrants	Bind bile in the gut	Reduce LDL	Cholestyramine	Diarrhea Constipation
Nicotinic acid	Activate adipocyte receptors	Reduce TG, LDL Increase HDL	Nicotinic acid (niacin)	Flushing Itching

Table 2.32 Cholesterol lowering medications.

bile acid sequestrants are not recommended but may be used in statin-intolerant patients.

Statins

Statins (e.g. simvastatin and atorvastatin) reduce cardio-vascular events and mortality in patients with CHD and re-

Clinical insight

Statins are metabolized in the liver by the cytochrome P450 (CYP3A4) enzyme system. Other chemicals that interfere with this (e.g. grapefruit, fibrates, niacin) lead to elevated levels of circulating statins.

duce the likelihood of CHD in those with hypercholesterolemia. They also improve endothelial function and maintain atherosclerotic plaque stability.

Other lipid-lowering drugs

Other drugs are generally not recommended in AHA/ACC or NICE guidelines for CHD prevention, but may be useful in some situations.

Fibrates There is no evidence that fibrates save lives in CHD, but they do reduce the risk of MI. They are used in patients intolerant to statins or in combination with statins when statin monotherapy is insufficient.

Brush border lipase inhibitors There is no evidence that brush border lipase inhibitors reduce cardiovascular mortality or morbidity. Ezetimibe is suggested by NICE as a second line therapy for familial hypercholesterolemia where patients are statin intolerant, or as combination therapy when statin monotherapy is isufficient.

Bile acid sequestrants Bile acid sequestrants, also known as anion exchange resins, reduce the progression of, and mortality in, CHD. They may be used as an accessory drug with statins, if fibrates are contraindicated.

Nicotinic acid The broad-spectrum effects of nicotinic acid reduce CHD mortality, but its clinical use is limited by a high rate of side effects such as flushing, rashes and GI upset.

Anti-coagulants

Anti-coagulants inhibit blood coagulation (**Figure 2.27** and **Table 2.33**).

Coumarins

Coumarins are taken orally to reduce venous thrombosis in DVT or PE, or prevent arterial thrombosis in patients with AF or metallic heart valves. For example, they reduce the risk of embolic stroke in patients with AF by 66%. The most widely used coumarin is warfarin. An initial dose (usually 5 or 10 mg daily) is given and daily blood tests monitor the patient's blood clotting, as measured by the international normalized ratio (INR). Once a target INR of 2–3 (ideally 2.5) is reached, a maintenance dose is continued and INR is monitored every 2–4 weeks to ensure a balance between clotting risk (e.g. MI or stroke risk) and bleeding risk.

Heparins

Heparins are natural glycosaminoglycans found in mast cells and basophils that inhibit thrombosis. Synthetic heparins

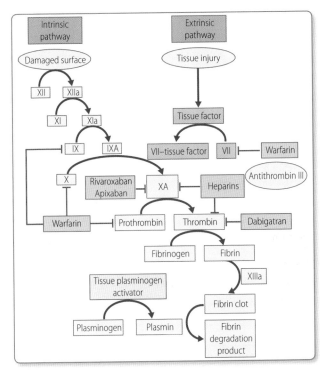

Figure 2.27 The clotting cascade and anti-coagulant drugs.

are used to prevent venous thrombosis in inpatients and the propagation of established thrombus in patients with DVT, PE or MI.

Low molecular weight heparins (LMWH), e.g. dalteparin and enoxaparin, are administered subcutaneously, whereas unfractionated heparin (UFH) is given as a continuous intravenous infusion.

Clinical insight

Heparin-induced thrombocytopenia (HIT) arises in 3–5% of patients following administration of heparin. Antibodies to heparin bind to platelets causing activation, clumping, reduced platelet count and subsequent (paradoxical) thrombosis.

Types and mode of action	Side effect	Antidote	Indications
COUMARINS: Inhibit clotting factors II, VII, IX, X, e.g. warfarin, phenindione	Bleeding Bruising Osteoporosis Hair loss	Vitamin K	AF VTE MHV
HEPARINS: Activate anti-thrombin III, e.g. enoxaparin dalteparin	Bleeding Bruising Hyperkalaemia Thrombocytopenia	Protamine sulphate	VTE MI
NOVEL ORAL ANTICOAGULANTS (NOACs): Inhibit thrombin directly, e.g. apixaban, rivaroxaban	Bleeding Bruising Headache Indigestion	N/A	VTE AF

AF, atrial fibrillation; MHV, metal heart valves; MI, myocardial infarction; VTE, venous thromboembolism.

Table 2.33 Anticoagulants.

Novel oral anticoagulants

Unlike warfarin, the novel oral anticoagulants (NOAC) such as dabigatran and rivaroxaban do not necessitate regular blood tests. They are approximately as effective as warfarin in a patient with DVT, PE or AF, and are used when warfarin is ineffective or when regular testing is difficult.

Anti-platelet drugs

Antiplatelet drugs (**Figure 2.28** and **Table 2.34**) inhibit platelet adhesion and aggregation and therefore thrombus formation. They are used in the primary prevention and treatment of thrombotic CHD and PVD. They are more effective in the arterial circulation.

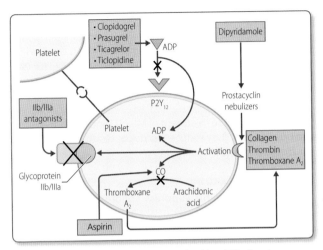

Figure 2.28 Mechanism of action of anti-platelet drugs. ADP, adenosine diphoshphate; COX, cyclo-oxygenase; GP IIb/IIIa, glycoprotein IIb/IIIa

Drug or drug group	Mode of action	Examples	Common side effects	Indications
Salicylic acid	Inhibits platelet cyclo-oxygenase (COX) enzyme	Aspirin	Bleeding Bruising Peptic ulceration Gout	CHD Cerebrovascular disease PVD
Thienopyridines	Inhibits platelet adenosine diphosphate (ADP)	Clopidogrel Prasugrel Ticagrelor	Bleeding Bruising Thrombocytopenia Dyspnea	MI Cerebrovascular disease PVD

Table 2.34 Anti-platelet medication. CHD, coronary heart disease; PVD, peripheral vascular disease; MI, myocardial infarction.

Salicylic acid

Salicylic acid (aspirin) is found in willow tree bark and many fruits. It is a minor analgesic and antipyretic, and is used as life-long antiplatelet treatment following diagnosis of CHD, PAD and MI. It reduces the risk of death in CHD by 30%.

Thienopyridines

These are used in the treatment of MI, PAD and cerebrovascular accidents (CVA). They reduce the risk of death and further MI by 20% in patients following MI.

Anti-arrhythmic drugs

Anti-arrhythmic agents suppress abnormal rhythms of the heart (**Table 2.35**).

Class I

Class I agents block the fast sodium channel of non-nodal cardiac myocytes which are responsible for the rapid depolarization (Phase 0) of the action potential.

Class II

Class II agents (beta-blockers) suppress atrial and ventricular arrhythmias, improve LV function in heart failure and reduce myocardial oxygen demand in CHD.

Mode of action Atenolol, bisoprolol and metoprolol antagonize β_1 adrenoreceptors, blocking sympathetic stimulation of the AVN. Carvedilol, labetalol, propranolol are non-selective and also target β_2 receptors causing bronchial muscle relaxation.

Class III

Class III agents (amiodarone and sotalol) are indicated in AF, ventricular tachycardia and ventricular fibrillation.

Mode of action These agents block cardiomyocyte potassium channels, lengthening the action potential and refractory period duration, preventing re-entrant arrhythmias.

Drug class	Mode of action	Effect on cardiac AP	Examples	Side effects	Indications in CHD
IA	Inhibit fast Na$^+$ channel	Lengthened	Procainamide Disopyramide	Diarrhea, nausea, headache, dizziness	N/A
IB		Shortened	Lidocaine Mexiletine	Dizziness, bradycardia, hypotension, arrhythmia, cardiac arrest	Ventricular tachycardia
IC		No effect	Flecainide Propafenone	Dizziness, nausea, dyspnea, arrhythmia	AF
II	Block β-adrenergic receptors	No effect	Bisoprolol Atenolol Propranolol	Bradycardia, heart block, bronchospasm, hyper/hypoglycemia, headache, constipation	Angina, AF, ventricular tachycardia, heart failure
III	Inhibit K$^+$ channel	Lengthened	Sotalol Amiodarone	Skin discoloration, thyroid dysfunction, corneal deposits, long QT	AF, ventricular tachycardia
IV	Blocks Ca^{2+} channels	Shortened	Diltiazem * Verapamil †	Bradycardia, hypotension, dizziness, and headache	AF, AFL, angina
V	Inhibits Na$^+$/K$^+$ ATPase	No effect	Digoxin	Anorexia, nausea, vomiting and tachy/bradyarrhythmias	Atrial fibrillation/flutter
	Transient AV block	No effect	Adenosine	Dyspnea, facial flushing, asystole, headache, apprehension	Supraventricular tachycardias

Table 2.35 Anti-arrhythmic medication: the Vaughn-Williams classification, based on effect on cardiac myocyte action potential. AP, action potential; AF, atrial fibrillation; AFL, atrial flutter. *A benzodiazepine. † A phenylalkylamine.

> ### Clinical insight
>
> Amiodarone has many side-effects, some are due to its structural similarity to thyroxine; a daily dose of amiodarone (200 mg) accounts for 20 times the daily requirement of thyroxine (6 mg).

Class IV

Class IV agents – calcium-channel blockers (CCB) – are used for atrial tachycardias and CHD.

Mode of action CCBs block all cardiac calcium channels to decrease the sinus rate and cardiac contractility, prolong the refractory period, and slow conduction through the AV node.

Class V

These are used for atrial tachycardias but have no common mechanism.

Adenosine Adenosine is a purine nucleoside that acts on the A1 receptor subtypes leading to cell hyperpolarization of both the SA and AV nodes, lengthening the refractory period. This temporarily blocks the AVN and prevents re-entry through the node, such as in SVT.

Digoxin Digoxin is a glycoside derived from foxglove (*Digitalis*) that inhibits the sodium/potassium adenosine triphosphate (ATP) pump in cardiac tissue. This increases intracellular sodium and calcium, slows SA and AVN conduction, and therefore ventricular contraction. It also augments cardiac contractility and is used in patients with heart failure.

Diuretics

Diuretics increase salt and water excretion (i.e. urine production) to lower blood pressure in hypertension and heart failure (**Figure 2.29** and **Table 2.36**). Most diuretics work by blocking different mechanisms of salt (Na^+ and/or K^+) reabsorption in the kidney.

Loop diuretics

Loop diuretics (e.g. furosemide) are the most powerful diuretics, leading to the excretion of 20% of filtered sodium. They are used to treat pulmonary and peripheral edema in heart failure, but do not reduce mortality.

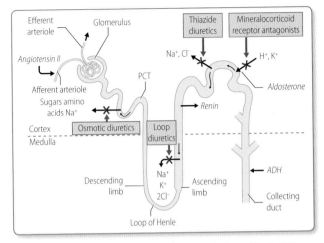

Figure 2.29 Diuretic drugs and their site of action at the loop of Henle. PCT, proximal convoluted tubule.

Thiazide diuretics

Thiazide diuretics (e.g. bendroflumethiazide) are used in hypertension to reduce blood pressure by an average of 10/5 mmHg.

Potassium sparing diuretics

'Potassium sparing' diuretics (e.g. amiloride) do not increase potassium loss in urine and are used in hypertension and heart failure, normally as adjuncts to other diuretics.

Mineralocorticoid receptor antagonists

Mineralocorticoid receptor/aldosterone antagonists (MRA's, e.g. spironolactone) are second-line potassium-sparing diuretics used in hypertension and heart failure. They reduce blood pressure by up to 17/10 mmHg and the risk of death by one third in patients with chronic severe heart failure.

MRAs also decrease cardiac hypertrophy, fibrosis and arrhythmias and improve endothelial function by an unknown mechanism.

Type of diuretic	Mode of action	Location of action	Examples	Common side effects	Indications
Loop	Block Na+/K+/Cl- cotransporter	Thick ascending limb	Furosemide Bumetanide	Hyponatremia Hypokalemia Hyperuricemia Renal injury	Heart failure
Thiazide	Block Na+/Cl- cotransporter	Distal convoluted tubule	Bendroflumethiazide Metolazone	Hypotension Dizziness Hyperglycemia Cholestasis	Heart failure Hypertension
Potassium sparing	Block epithelial Na+ channels	Collecting duct	Amiloride Triamterene	Hyperkalemia Dizziness Rash	Hypertension
Mineralocorticoid receptor antagonists	Block aldosterone receptors	Distal convoluted tubule	Spironolactone Eplerenone	Breast tenderness Hyperkalaemia	Heart failure Hypertension

Table 2.36 Diuretics. CHD, coronary heart disease.

Anti-hypertensives

Antihypertensives lower systemic vascular resistance, and therefore blood pressure, in primary and secondary prevention of CHD and CVAs (**Table 2.37**).

Alpha-blockers

Alpha-blockers (e.g. doxazo-sin) are first-line agents that can decrease blood pressure by 11/7 mmHg. They block

> **Clinical insight**
>
> Alpha-blockers should be avoided in heart failure as they increase mortality.

noradrenaline (norepinephrine) binding to alpha-1 adreno-receptors in vascular smooth muscle, leading to dilation of arteries and veins.

Angiotensin converting enzyme inhibitors

Angiotensin converting enzyme (ACE) inhibitors (**Figure 2.30**) are first-line treatments of hypertension, heart failure, diabetic nephropathy and following MI. They reduce the risk of MI and CVAs by 11% in hypertension. Following MI, they reduce the risk of death and heart failure by 25%, by reducing cardiac hypertrophy, progression of heart failure and proteinuria.

Angiotensin II receptor blockers

Angiotensin II receptor blockers (ARBs) are second-line agents used in hypertension and heart failure (**Figure 2.30**). They reduce the risk of MI by 10% in hypertension and death by 25% in severe heart failure, by reducing cardiac hypertrophy, progression of heart failure and proteinuria.

Hydralazine

Hydralazine is a second-line agent in hypertension and heart failure. It can reduce blood pressure by up to 25/17 mmHg and mortality

> **Clinical insight**
>
> ACEIs cause a dry tickly cough in 20% due to build up of lung bradykinin, a peptide that causes pulmonary irritation and bronchoconstriction.

in heart failure by 25%. It stimulates calcium release from the sarcoplasmic reticulum, leading to vasodilation, reduction of systemic vascular resistance and blood pressure.

Drug	Mode of action	Examples	Common side effect	Indications in CHD
Alpha-blockers	Block α-1 adrenoreceptors	Doxazosin	Dizziness Urinary incontinence Hypotension	Hypertension
Angiotensin converting enzyme inhibitors	Block conversion of angiotensin I to angiotensin II	Ramipril Enalapril Lisinopril	Dry cough Hyperkalemia Renal injury Angio-edema	Hypertension Heart failure Diabetic nephropathy Myocardial infarction
Angiotensin II receptor blockers	Block angiotensin II AT1 receptor	Valsartan Candesartan Losartan	Dizziness Hyperkalemia Renal injury Angio-edema	Hypertension Heart failure Diabetic nephropathy Myocardial infarction
Hydralazine	Direct peripheral vasodilation	Hydralazine	Allergic reaction Drug induced lupus Palpitations	Hypertension Heart failure
Calcium channel blockers	Block L-type calcium channels	Amlodipine Felodipine Nifedipine	Dizziness Flushing Ankle/gum swelling	Hypertension CHD

Table 2.37 Antihypertensives. AT, angiotensin; CHD, coronary heart disease.

Figure 2.30 The mechanism of action of angiotensin converting enzyme inhibitors (ACEIs) and angiotensin II receptor blockers (ARBs). ACEIs block ACE converting angiotensin I (ATI) to angiotensin II (ATII) leading to inhibition of the renin-angiotensin-aldosterone system (RAAS). Less AT II leads to peripheral dilation, reducing cardiac pre and afterload, improving endothelial function, reducing sympathetic tone and reducing blood pressure. ARBs inhibit the RAAS by blocking the AT1 receptor of ATII leading to arteriolar and venous dilation. ARBs reduce cardiac pre and afterload, improve endothelial function, reduce sympathetic tone and blood pressure. JGA, juxtaglomerular apparatus.

Calcium channel blockers (dihydropyridines)

The dihydropyridines are first-line agents to treat hypertension, and second-line in CHD, reducing blood pressure by 13/11 mmHg and the risk of MI by 11%, respectively. CCBs inhibit L-type calcium channels in vascular smooth muscle, causing arterial vasodilation, decreasing peripheral resistance and improving coronary perfusion.

Anti-anginal drugs

Nitrates, beta-blockers and calcium-channel blockers are the first line treatment of angina (**Table 2.38**).

Clinical insight

Calcium channel blockers can exacerbate pulmonary and peripheral edema.

Nitrates

Nitrates are a first-line treatment of angina, hypertensive crises, acute coronary syndromes and acute heart failure. In patients intolerant to ACEI, they are used in conjunction with hydralazine in chronic heart failure, leading to a 34% reduction in mortality.

Mode of action These are precursors to nitric oxide, a powerful localized venous and arterial vasodilator that reduces cardiac

Types and mode of action	Common side effects	Indications
FIRST LINE		
Nitric oxide donor; e.g. GTN, isosorbide	Headaches Dizziness Hypotension	CHD
SECOND LINE		
Nitric oxide donor and potassium channel agonist, e.g. Nicorandil	Palpitations Flushing Gastric ulcers	CHD HF MI
Funny channel agonist, e.g. ivabradine	Flashing lights Bradycardia Dizziness	CHD
Sodium channel blocker, e.g. ranolazine	Palpitations Long QT Indigestion	CHD

Table 2.38 Anti-anginal medication. CHD, coronary heart disease; GTN, glyceryl trinitrate; HF, heart failure; MI, myocardial infarction.

preload, afterload, myocardial oxygen demand and blood pressure. Side effects include headaches, dizziness, nausea, vomiting and hypotension.

Nicorandil

Nicorandil is a second-line anti-anginal agent and is a nitric oxide precursor. Usage results in a 15% reduction in MI.

Ivabradine

This is a second-line anti-anginal agent used in patients with normal sinus rhythm and heart rate >70 bpm. It reduces the risk of MI by 33% but doesn't reduce mortality. Ivabradine blocks the funny channel in the SA node, reducing heart rate.

Ranolazine

This is used to treat angina, likely by blocking the sodium dependent calcium channels. It has minimal effect on blood pressure and heart rate and no impact on MI or mortality, but reduces anginal episodes by 1–2 per week.

2.7 Surgical management

Cardiovascular surgery is often high-risk, necessitating objective measures of risk before, during and after surgery: risk score, co-morbidity, functional status and cardiovascular fitness.

Percutaneous coronary intervention

In percutaneous coronary intervention (PCI), also known as angioplasty, a balloon is used to widen the lumen of a coronary artery narrowed by atheroma and stabilize the plaque (**Figure 2.31**).

Complications   These include:
- MI – 3%
- Coronary dissection – 3%
- Death – 3%
- Stroke – 1%

Arterial bypass

Arterial bypass uses a synthetic or transplanted vessel to circumvent a section of blocked artery. It is indicated in patients with

Figure 2.31 Percutaneous coronary intervention (PCI). (a) The stent is crimped over the balloon and guide wire. (b) Inflating the balloon expands the stent. (c) The stent in situ.

Clinical insight

Stents can be bare metal (cobalt–chromium alloy) or coated with drugs, such as sirolimus or paclitaxel, that prevent cell proliferation and thrombosis.

significant atherosclerotic lesions, particularly left main stem and triple coronary vessel.

Procedure A coronary artery bypass graft (CABG; **Figure 2.32**) is performed under general anesthetic and takes approximately 4 hours:

- the chest is opened via midline sternal incision (median sternotomy) a cardiopulmonary bypass is established with a heart lung machine (90 minutes) 'cardioplegia' – the heart is cooled with iced salt water, while a preservative solution is injected into the heart arteries
- The grafts are harvested (**Table 2.39**), washed and sewn proximal to the blockage, typically the aorta, and to the coronary artery distal to the blockage
- The patient is taken off bypass, the chest closed with wires and anesthetic reversed

Complications These include:

- Death – <1%
- Bleeding – 2%

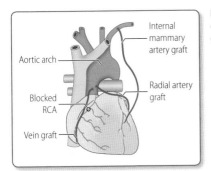

Figure 2.32 A triple coronary artery bypass graft.

Internal mammary artery graft

Aortic arch

Blocked RCA

Radial artery graft

Vein graft

	Venous graft	**Arterial graft**
Example	Long saphenous vein of leg	Internal mammary of thorax
Length	Long	Limited
10 year patency	66%	90%

Table 2.39 Venous versus arterial coronary artery bypass grafts. Venous grafts are more prone to stenosis and deteriorate within 7 years in approximately half of patients.

- Thromboembolism – 1%
- Infection – 4%
- Myocardial infarction – 5%
- Temporary arrhythmias (e.g. AF) – 25%

Arterial repair

Abnormal dilations, acute dissections and focal atherosclerosis of large arteries, such as an AAA (> 5.5 cm) or carotid atherosclerosis (50–99%), are repaired under general anesthetic.

Procedure For a carotid endarterectomy, for example:
- An incision is made over the carotid artery and a clamp placed above and below the blockage
- The artery is cut open and the atherosclerotic lesion removed
- The skin is closed and the anesthetic reversed.

Heart transplantation

Heart transplantation is a life-saving treatment for end-stage heart disease.

Procedure Following a general anesthetic:
- The chest is opened via midline sternal incision (median sternotomy)
- The patient is put on a bypass machine
- The heart is isolated from the major vessels and removed
- The donor heart is implanted and sewn to the vessels
- Finally, the patient is taken off the bypass machine, the chest is closed and the anesthetic is reversed.

> ### Clinical insight
> Heart transplantation is limited by availability, e.g. around 200 were performed in the UK in 2013.

Complications Complications include death, stroke, bleeding, thromboembolism, transplant failure, infection, myocardial infarction and cardiac arrhythmia.

Valve repair/replacement

This is indicated in patients with symptomatic and severe valve disease not amenable to minimally invasive repair.

Procedure Following a general anesthetic:
- The chest is opened via midline sternal incision (median sternotomy)
- The patient is put on a bypass machine and then the heart is then cooled
- The diseased valve is located and removed
- For repair of the mitral valve, stitches are used to repair the prolapsing leaflet and secure it to the valvular apparatus
- For replacement, a new tissue or metal valve is then sewn into place
- The patient is taken off bypass, the chest is closed and the anesthetic reversed.

Complications The complications include death, stroke, bleeding, thromboembolism, valve dehiscence, infection, myocardial infarction and cardiac arrhythmia.

Procedure	Indication	Purpose	Method
Left ventricular assist device	LV failure pre-transplant or post MI	Assist myocardial recovery	Pump inlet is sewn to the LV apex and the pump outlet to the ascending aorta
Total artificial heart	End-stage heart failure	Complete replacement of heart function	Cardiac chambers are removed and the device attached to the great vessels
LV restoration therapy	LV aneurysm post-MI	Improves LV function	Diseased myocardium removed and the heart then closed
Septal repair	ASD, VSD, If septum cannot be closed using a device	Separation of left and right circulation	Patch of bovine/native pericardium or Teflon is sewn into place

Table 2.40 Examples of myocardial repair and support.

Myocardial repair and support

Certain myocardial defects are suitable for repair and/or the failing myocardium can be supported by use of an artificial pump (Table 2.40).

Atherosclerosis

Atherosclerosis is a progressive process of atheroma formation – arterial wall lesions of white blood cells, lipid and cholesterol deposits and cell debris. These 'plaques' form in the intima of large and medium arteries, and can develop to include scar tissue, thrombosis and calcification.

All larger arteries develop atheroma as we age, but in excess it can cause hardening of the arterial wall (sclerosis) and narrowing of the lumen. The resulting obstruction restricts blood flow to cause ischemia of downstream tissues. If the plaque becomes unstable and ruptures, thrombosis and thromboembolism can cause acute blockage and infarction of tissue.

Atherosclerosis is the underlying cause of most coronary and cerebral arterial disease; the two biggest killers in the western world. It is also accelerated by diabetes mellitus and underlies most peripheral vascular disease.

3.1 Clinical scenario

Painful, cold right foot
Presentation
Carol Newton is a 56-year-old store manager who presents to her local emergency department with a painful and cold right foot.

Diagnostic approach
Foot pain is common and causes include peripheral vascular disease (PVD), gout, plantar fasciitis and ligament sprain. However, a cold foot suggests a problem with the blood supply. History should establish:

- Onset
- If it is worsening
- Associated symptoms, such as numbness and radiation of pain.

Clinical insight

The symptoms of acute limb ischemia are the six P's.

- Pain
- Pulseless
- Pallor
- Perishingly cold
- Paresthesia
- Paralysis

Further history

The pain has been increasing for a couple of days, was not preceded by trauma, and has no focal tender point. It is worse when she lies in bed, causing her to hang her foot out of the bed. She is a lifelong smoker but has no other significant past medical history and takes no medications.

Examination

Other than having blood pressure of 155/95 mmHg, Carol's cardiovascular, respiratory and abdominal systems are all normal. She is afebrile, has normal oxygen saturation and blood glucose.

Her right foot is pale and pulseless, with a delayed capillary refill time of 6 s. The most distally palpable pulse is the femoral artery. Dorsiflexion and plantar flexion are difficult and painful when done passively.

Diagnostic approach

Lack of trauma or focal tenderness suggests the pain is unlikely to originate from the musculoskeletal system or a single structure. Night pain is common in lower limb ischemia, because the raised limb decreases blood flow; lowering the foot increases flow and decreases the ischemic pain.

Smoking and hypertension are major risk factors for atherosclerosis, increasing the likelihood of PVD. Accordingly, her delayed capillary refill time suggests impaired blood supply due to either the heart or the arteries.

The normal oxygen saturation, blood glucose and temperature rule out hypoxia, hyperglycemia, hypothermia or overt sepsis as contributing factors, respectively. Cardiogenic or septic shock is unlikely as only one limb is affected and she isn't hypotensive.

A unilateral pulseless and cold foot confirms an arterial etiology, likely distal to her palpable femoral artery.

Investigations

An electrocardiogram (ECG) and further blood tests (including full blood count and tests of renal and liver function) are done and are all normal.

The ankle−brachial pressure index (ABPI) is <0.5 (75 mmHg/155 mmHg).

Diagnosis

The diagnosis is acute lower limb ischemia, as indicated by the unilateral painful, cold and pulseless foot and ABPI of <0.5, confirming a significantly lower blood pressure in her right foot than her arms. The foot pain at rest and delayed capillary refill indicate that tissue viability is threatened. Her difficulty in moving the foot means that urgent revascularization is necessary.

The blood tests are performed to obtain pre-operative baseline values as blood loss and significant organ injury may follow any limb or life-saving operation.

Carol's condition is likely due to peripheral arterial atherosclerosis caused by cigarette smoking and worsened by uncontrolled hypertension.

> ### Clinical insight
>
> Patients with peripheral arterial disease are at higher risk of CHD and cerebrovascular disease.

3.2 Atherosclerosis

Atherosclerosis is the most common arterial pathology and underlies most disease of ischemia and infarction. Its features depend on the site affected, resulting from arterial constriction at the lesion and embolic disease. Treatment can be symptomatic relief of vasoconstriction, surgical removal of a thrombus, and stabilization or bypass of the plaque. Primary and/or secondary prevention aims to treat symptoms and decrease risk factors.

Epidemiology

Atheroma begins to form as fatty streaks in late childhood, and progresses with age. By the 8th or 9th decades, all medium and larger arteries have some degree of atheroma.

Atherosclerosis causes more deaths than any other pathophysiology.

Non-modifiable risk factors include age, sex and genetic predisposition (**Table 3.1**). Symptomatic disease is most common in males over 40.

Etiology

The lipid-rich, inflammatory cell and debris deposits of atheroma are a part of normal aging (**Figure 3.1**). However, the process is accelerated in individuals with a family history of coronary artery disease or stroke, hyperlipidemia, diabetes mellitus, smoking and hypertension.

Guiding principle

Athere- is from a Greek word for 'gruel', a reference to the gross appearance of atheroma. 'Sclerosis' is from the word *skleros* meaning 'hard', describing the hardened fibrous cap of plaques.

Location

Hemodynamics – the physical forces of blood flow – affects where plaques tend to occur. Branched or curved sections of arteries, or areas where blood flow changes velocity or direction, are prone to atheroma. These areas have non-laminar flow with associated low shear stress, which promotes endothelial dysfunction and monocyte infiltration. Atheroma occurs most in the aorta, followed by the carotid, coronary, and iliofemoral arteries.

Prevention

Prevention focuses on reducing modifiable risk factors with changes in lifestyle and medications (see Chapter 9). Lifestyle changes include cessation of smoking, regular exercise, weight loss if obese and control of diabetes and hypertension. A healthy diet is low in fat – especially saturated fat – salt, sugar, cholesterol, alcohol and high in fresh fruit and vegetables – and therefore antioxidants – and fiber.

Aggressive lowering of LDL cholesterol can delay, stall and possibly even reverse atherogenesis.

Risk factor	Definition	Mechanism
Smoking	Tobacco smoke	Provokes endothelial damage and thrombosis
High blood cholesterol	Age, sex, heredity, and diet affect cholesterol High total cholesterol >6.2 mmol/L (240 mg/dL) High LDL cholesterol >3.4 mmol/L (130 mg/dL)	Increases cholesterol deposition in arterial wall
High triglycerides	>4.5 mmol/L (400 mg/dL)	Increases lipid deposition in arterial wall
Hypertension	>140/90 mmHg	Provokes endothelial damage
Physical inactivity	>4 hours siting a day, <30 min exercise 4 times a week	Increases thrombosis and exposure of vascular endothelium to glucose, lipids and toxins and decreases cardiovascular muscle fitness
Diabetes mellitus	Most diabetics die from myocardial infarction secondary to atherosclerosis	Hyperglycemia promotes endothelial and vascular connective tissue damage
Stress	History	Increased heart rate, blood pressure and circulating leukocytes
Obesity	BMI >30 kg/m^2	Increases vascular workload

Table 3.1 Risk factors for atherosclerosis and their contributory mechanism.

Pathogenesis

Atherogenesis is generally considered a disordered response to endothelial injury, involving interactions between vascular endothelium, macrophages, smooth muscle cells, leukocytes and platelets (**Figures 3.1** and **3.2**).

1. Endothelial injury occurs due to oxidized LDL, infections, toxins, free radical damage, hyperglycemia or hyper-homocystinemia, amongst others

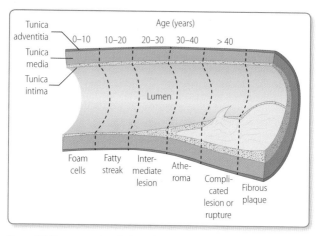

Figure 3.1 The progression of atherosclerosis.

Figure 3.2
Hematoxylin and eosin staining of coronary artery (right) and vein (left). The artery shows a markedly diminished lumen (1) due to atherosclerotic plaque on the right side. There is a fibrous cap (2) overlying necrotic core matrix and cholesterol crystals (3). Some calcification is also present (4). Support fibrofatty tissue (5). Courtesy of Dr S.K. Suvarna.

2. Vascular inflammation – monocytes in the blood adhere to and pass through the endothelium to infiltrate the arterial tunica intima and become macrophages, responsible for digesting debris and bacteria

3. Foam cell formation and accumulation – macrophages consume oxidized LDL cholesterol to form foam cells, which promote inflammation (**Figure 3.3**)

4. Foam cells proliferate to form the fatty streak – also known as intimal xanthoma – appearance of early atherosclerosis, along with T cells and smooth muscle cells

5. Fibroproliferation occurs as activated smooth muscle cells and recruited fibroblasts produce extracellular matrix, i.e. scar tissue

6. Scar tissue forms a fibrous plaque on the lumen side, covering the foam cells and deposits of lipid and necrotic cellular debris

7. The plaque grows, stimulating neovascularization of fragile vessels, and increasingly occluding the lumen.

Atherogenesis is generally progressive, but with periods of quiescence. Although it is a systemic disease, it manifests, usually at a late stage, with focal signs and symptoms. Symptoms develop as ischemia progresses, or occur acutely with plaque rupture or erosion, which can be catastrophic.

Plaque rupture Acute complications occur if the plaque ruptures or bleeds, promoting thrombosis and thromboembolism that can partially or completely block the artery (**Figure 3.4**). Rupture is predisposed by structurally unstable fibrous caps and increasing size of the necrotic core. It is also associated with

- Neovascularizaton
- Intra-plaque hemorrhage/iron deposition in the lesion.
- The presence of inflammatory enzymes
- Non-laminar blood flow
- Macrophage calcification.

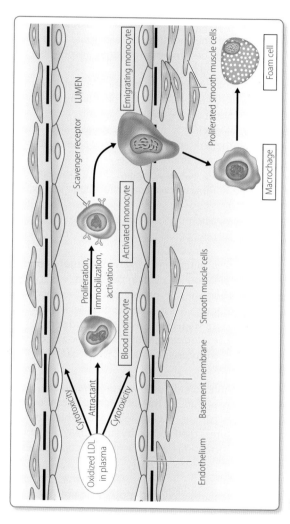

Figure 3.3 The formation of foam cells – the initiation of atherogenesis.

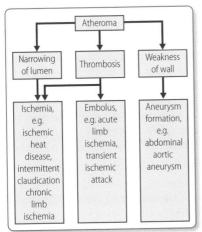

Figure 3.4 Complications of atherosclerosis.

Atherosclerosis also weakens vascular connective tissue, increasing the risk of aneurysm formation and associated wall rupture.

Plaque erosion Acute arterial occlusion can also occur when endothelium covering or near the plaque erodes to expose smooth muscle cells and extra-cellular matrix. This initiates the clotting cascade and thrombosis, which can block the vessel at the lesion site or distally by thrombo-embolism.

Guiding principle

Vascular endothelial cells have important roles in atherogenesis, as key regulators of:

- Hemostasis, by secreting antithrombotic (e.g. heparin sulphate) and, under stress, prothrombotic molecules
- Blood flow, by secretion of vasodilators, e.g. prostacyclin and nitrous oxide, and when activated, vasoconstrictors (e.g. endothelin)
- The immune response – when stimulated by injury, they attract leukocytes with chemokines and express surface adhesion molecules to allow entry to the vascular wall.

Immune dysregulation   Vascular injury activates smooth muscle cells and endothelial cells to express inflammatory mediators, vasoactive compounds and surface adhesion molecules to recruit immune cells, i.e. monocytes/macrophages lymphocytes, dendritic antigen-presenting cells and fibroblasts. This immune response is dysregulated in atherosclerosis.

The involvement of immune cells means there is some overlap with diseases of immune dysregulation, such as autoimmune disease. For example, continually raised levels of C-reactive protein are predictive of symptomatic peripheral vascular disease in later life.

Calcification   As plaque cells die, calcium deposits crystallize and collect at the border between the plaque and vascular smooth muscle. This intramural calcification occurs as plaques age, decreasing elasticity of the wall. In late stages, calcifications are seen on CT images as halos of increased radiodensity around atheromatous plaques.

Clinical features

Atherosclerosis can occur in any medium or large artery and is mostly asymptomatic. It causes signs and symptoms by obstruction of blood flow at the site of atheroma or acute thromboembolic occlusion downstream (**Table 3.2**). Lesions increase the risk of aneurysm or dissection of an artery. For example, an abdominal aortic aneurysm presents as an asymptomatic pulsatile abdominal mass, but is at increasing risk of rupture and massive hemorrhage as it increases in size.

Ischemic pain, such as leg claudication or angina, increases proportional to exertion, as the metabolic needs of tissues are not met by the limited blood supply. Conversely, it improves on rest.

Lesions may be evident on palpation as pulsatile, hardened masses, and bruits heard on auscultation due to turbulent blood flow.

All patients should be assessed for features of atherosclerotic risk factors, as most disease is asymptomatic and prevention is based on control of modifiable risk factors (**Table 3.3**).

Site	Ischemic pathology	Infarcted pathology
Coronary arteries	Angina	Myocardial infarction
Carotid arteries	Transient ischemic attack	Hemorrhagic or ischemic cerebrovascular accident
Cerebral arteries		
Iliofemoral arteries	Intermittent claudication	Impotence, persistent ulceration and infection of peripheries, necrosis, gangrene
Mesenteric arteries	Mesenteric angina – epigastric postprandial pain	Hematemesis, hematochezia, diarrhea, melena, nutritional deficiencies, and weight loss
Renal arteries	Renal artery stenosis; resistant hypertension	Kidney atrophy, necrosis, renal failure

Table 3.2 The site of atherosclerosis and associated features of ischemic and infarcted pathology.

Risk factor	Clinical features
Smoking	History; tar-stained fingers or hair
High blood cholesterol/triglycerides	Xanthelasma and tendon xanthoma
Hypertension	BP >140/90 mmHg
Sedentary lifestyle	History, overweight or obese
Diabetes mellitus	History, raised blood glucose or HbA1c
Obesity	BMI >30 kg/m^2

Table 3.3 The main clinical features of risk factors for atherosclerosis.

Diagnostic approach

Diagnosis involves assessing for atherosclerotic risk factors, imaging of arteries to visualize lesions and loss of lumen patency, stress testing to indicate loss of blood flow

Clinical insight

Atherosclerosis is a systemic disease; evidence of it in one artery usually indicates its presence in other arteries. For example, peripheral vascular disease strongly suggests there are similar lesions in the coronary arteries.

as well as assessment of end organ damage due to ischemia or infarction.

Investigations

Atherosclerotic disease is investigated with blood tests to assess for risk factors or signs of end organ damage, imaging to visualize the lesion and functional tests that gauge the ischemic effect of the lesion.

Laboratory tests A lipid profile assesses for hyperlipidemia; high levels of LDL cholesterol are associated with increased atherosclerosis. Blood glucose and hemoglobin A_{1c} (HbA_{1c}) are measured to monitor for diabetes.

Some blood tests, such as cardiac enzymes, can indicate the timing and extent of tissue ischemia or infarct. A raised white blood cell count is often found post myocardial infarction.

Imaging Doppler ultrasound is used to quantify the extent of atherosclerotic stenosis in the carotid arteries (see page 138). Angiography (see page 137) can be performed in cerebral, coronary, peripheral, mesenteric or renal arteries to visualize the extent of narrowing. As contrast is injected into the circulation, the lumen is visible on X-ray, CT or MRI. CT is usually best as it is high resolution and quicker to perform than MRI.

CT calcium scoring quantifies the amount of calcification present within the coronary circulation, which correlates with plaque size (see page 142). It does not show areas of soft plaque or thrombus.

Imaging can be essential for diagnosing and assessing end organ damage from infarction. For example, a CT of the head is essential to investigate a suspected cerebrovascular accident.

Functional testing Stress testing, such as the cardiac stress test, is used to assess the significance of a coronary stenosis and can indicate loss of function due to ischemia.

Management

Primary and secondary prevention focuses on control of risk factors, including lifestyle changes and medication.

Symptomatic treatment, such as glyceryl trinitrate, relieves ischemic pain. Revascularization of the circulation is either by percutaneous intervention using stents or bypass surgery (see page 163).

Lifestyle Lifestyle changes reduce or control modifiable risk factors and are central to primary and secondary prevention (see Chapter 9):
- Smoking cessation
- Strict control of hypertension and diabetes
- Regular aerobic exercise, i.e. >30 min/day most days of the week
- A Mediterranean-style diet, rich in fresh fruit and vegetables.

The widespread incidence means all patients should be encouraged to meet these targets, which also benefit general health and wellbeing.

As disease remains asymptomatic until a late stage, patients can be motivated by discussion of cardiovascular or cerebrovascular risk scores (see page 145), and referral to fitness training, dieticians or other specialists.

Medication Common medications include those to manage hyperlipidemia, hypertension, diabetes mellitus and smoking cessation.

Surgery Surgical treatments are indicated for patients with ongoing symptoms despite optimal medical management.

Prognosis

Atherosclerosis is a multifactorial disease with a genetic predisposition but lifestyle plays an equally important

> **Clinical insight**
>
> Venous grafts used in heart bypass surgery also develop atherosclerosis.

role. Patients present in many different ways and symptoms do not clearly correlate with the level of atherosclerosis. Some patients remain asymptomatic throughout life, while for others the first sign may be sudden cardiac death.

Although primary prevention and medical and surgical symptomatic treatments are improving, there is no direct treatment of the underlying disease.

Hypertension

Hypertension is chronically and abnormally high arterial blood pressure.

Hypertension is the major risk factor for coronary heart disease (CHD), peripheral vascular disease (PVD) and cerebrovascular disease, by damaging arteries to cause arterial wall inflammation and atherogenesis. Globally, CHD causes a third of all deaths, and hypertension is believed to be responsible for at least 50% of these.

Most hypertension is primary (i.e. 'essential'), a result of multiple genetic and environmental factors that increase peripheral vascular resistance. Secondary causes include renal artery, vascular and endocrine disease.

As it is largely asymptomatic, diagnosis depends on regular opportunistic screenings.

4.1 Clinical scenario

Opportunistic blood pressure measurement

Presentation

Janet Johnson, aged 57 years, visits her primary care doctor for an annual review of her type 2 diabetes mellitus. Her doctor measures her blood pressure twice:

- 167/98 mmHg
- 170/95 mmHg.

Diagnostic approach

Two blood pressure readings >140/90 mmHg indicate that Janet has hypertension. As she also has diabetes, she is at increased risk of CHD, PVD and cerebrovascular disease.

Further history

Janet is an office worker with a sedentary lifestyle. She eats processed foods, but little fresh fruit and vegetables. She smokes 20 cigarettes a day and drinks about 35 units of alcohol most weekends.

Her uncle and father both died from heart attacks in their late fifties.

Examination

Cardiovascular examination is normal except for her high body mass index (BMI) of 33 kg/m^2. Dipstick urinalysis shows glycosuria and proteinuria. Fundoscopic examination excludes signs of hypertensive retinopathy (see page 123).

Diagnostic approach

It is clear from her family history, diabetes, smoking, poor diet, lack of exercise and age that Janet has a significant risk of cardiovascular disease, but investigations are indicated to establish a diagnosis, estimate her total cardiovascular risk and assess for end organ damage:

1. Ambulatory blood pressure monitoring (ABPM) for 24 hours for a more accurate assessment of her blood pressure
2. Lipid profile to assess for hyperlipidemia
3. Kidney function tests including creatinine clearance or estimated glomerular filtration rate (eGFR) to assess for diabetic or hypertensive damage to glomerular blood vessels – either might be causing her proteinuria
4. Heart function: A 12-lead electrocardiogram (ECG) is indicated to look for evidence of left ventricular hypertrophy (LVH) and signs of IHD.

Fundoscopy is the easiest assessment of end-organ damage, and this was negative in her case.

Investigations

Janet returns a week later with her results (Table 4.1). These, along with her age, gender, diabetic status, smoking status and activity level are entered in the European Society of Cardiology HeartScore on-line cardiovascular risk calculator, which estimates her 10-year risk of death, stroke or heart attack to be 43%.

Diagnosis

In view of her age and the lack of suspicious symptoms or signs, there is no need to investigate further for secondary causes; the diagnosis is essential hypertension. Although her 10-year

Test	Result
24 h ABPM	152/93 mmHg
ECG	Normal sinus rhythm
Urea and electrolytes	All in normal range
eGFR	82 mL/min/1.73 m^2
Total cholesterol	5.8 mmol/L (224 mg/dL)
HDL cholesterol	1.16 mmol/L (44.8 mg/dL)

Table 4.1 Janet's results. ABPM, ambulatory blood pressure monitoring; ECG, electrocardiography; eGFR, estimated glomerular filtration rate; HDL, high-density lipoprotein.

risk is high, if her systolic blood pressure is normalized to 120 mmHg, her risk decreases to 32%. If she also stops smoking, becomes more active and reduces her total cholesterol to <5.2 mmol/L (200.7 mg/dL), this reduces to 17%.

Clinical insight

Online cardiovascular risk calculators use data from a large population but are only an estimate of an individual's cardiovascular risk. They can be a powerful clinical tool to help convey the benefits of treatment to an asymptomatic patient.

A combination of lifestyle changes and drug therapy is required to reduce her blood pressure and the risk of IHD, cerebrovascular disease, end organ damage and premature death.

4.2 Essential hypertension

Essential hypertension – also known as primary or idiopathic hypertension – is an increased systemic blood pressure in the absence of any identifiable pathological cause. It accounts for approximately 95% of all cases of hypertension, with the remaining 5% due to secondary hypertension.

It is important to be aware of local guidelines as definitions of hypertension as well as, diagnostic criteria and treatment protocols vary.

Types

Hypertension is widely defined as a persistent systolic blood pressure of over 140 mmHg, a diastolic blood pressure over 90 mmHg, or both. Ideal blood pressure is under 120/80 mmHg. A systolic pressure between 120–140 mmHg and a diastolic 80–90 mmHg are considered 'high-normal'.

Hypertension severity is graded into stages (**Table 4.2**) to inform the treatment strategy, as the risk of cardiovascular events is proportional to severity. Overall cardiovascular risk also depends on the presence of other risk factors (**Table 4.3**).

Epidemiology

Hypertension is a global problem. Risk factors are associated with a western lifestyle (**Table 4.3**), but hypertension is most prevalent in low- and middle-income countries due to recent urbanization (**Figure 4.1**).

African-Caribbean populations have a higher prevalence of hypertension than white and Asian populations due to a genetic tendency towards low renin levels, increased sensitivity to salt and impairment of salt excretion. Furthermore, people

Condition	Systolic blood pressure (mmHg)	Diastolic blood pressure (mmHg)
Ideal	<120	<80
High normal hypertension	120–139	80–89
Stage 1 hypertension	140–159	90–99
Stage 2 hypertension	160–179	100–109
Stage 3 hypertension	≥180	≥110
Accelerated hypertension	Same as stage 3 hypertension but with signs of grade 3 or 4 retinopathy	

Table 4.2 The stages of hypertension. Precise boundaries differ depending on the methods and guideline used. Repeated elevated measurements are needed to establish a diagnosis of hypertension as outlined in Figure 4.2.

	Risk factor	Mechanism
Modifiable	Obesity	Multifactorial, but obesity is associated with increased activity of the sympathetic nervous system, renin, angiotensinogen, angiotensin II and aldosterone
	Increased salt intake	Increased salt intake increases serum osmolality, which triggers increased water retention and peripheral vasoconstriction
	Excessive alcohol intake	Chronic excessive alcohol consumption is associated with hypertension, but the mechanism is not fully understood
	Sedentary lifestyle	Regular aerobic exercise is associated with healthier blood pressure
	Nicotine (smoking)	Nicotine causes increased cardiac output and peripheral vasoconstriction
Non-modifiable	Family history of hypertension	Multifactorial and heterogenous, but there is a polygenic influence
	Advanced age	Reduced arterial compliance
	African-Caribbean heritage	Reduced renin, increased sensitivity of blood pressure to salt and impairment of salt excretion all result in expansion of blood volume
	Male gender (<50 years)	Men and women are equal overall but men are affected at a younger age, possibly due to excess of other risk factors

Table 4.3 Modifiable and non-modifiable risk factors for essential hypertension.

of African descent have a greater tendency to develop cardio-vascular disease, especially stroke.

Etiology
Essential hypertension is due to multiple factors that cause widespread constriction of arterioles and small arteries which increases peripheral vascular resistance. Hypertension is more common in those with affected family members and multiple genes are implicated.

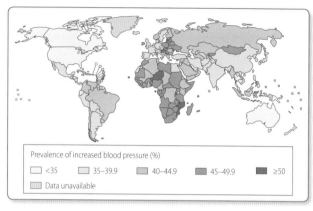

Prevalence of increased blood pressure (%)

☐ <35   ☐ 35–39.9   ☐ 40–44.9   ☐ 45–49.9   ☐ ≥50

☐ Data unavailable

Figure 4.1 The global burden of hypertension. High-income countries have a lower prevalence of hypertension, and low- and middle-income countries have a higher prevalence. Raised blood pressure is defined as a systolic blood pressure ≥140 mmHg and diastolic blood pressure ≥90 mmHg or using medication to lower blood pressure. Redrawn with permission from World Health Organization (WHO). Raised blood pressure, 2008. Geneva: WHO, 2008. http://gamapserver. who.int/gho/interactive_charts/ncd/risk_factors/blood_pressure_prevalence/ atlas.html. (Last accessed June 2014.)

Factors may include genetic, environmental or even behavioral traits that affect blood pressure regulation. Factors that affect the renin-angiotensin-aldosterone system (RAAS; see page 62) are particularly important. As hypertension progresses, excessive activation of sympathetic (adrenergic) nerves and the RAAS is usually seen.

Clinical insight

The history and examination should be tailored to the individual patient. For example, signs of aortic coarctation should be sought in a young patient with severe upper body hypertension, but essential hypertension is far more likely in an 80-year-old with high overall cardiovascular risk.

Clinical features

Blood pressure should be measured whenever possible to detect hypertension as it is usually asymptomatic unless severe. Diagnosis requires multiple careful readings (**Figure 4.2**).

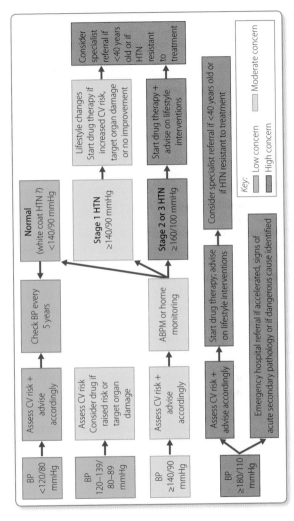

Figure 4.2 Diagnosis, investigation and management of hypertension. ABPM, ambulatory BP monitoring; HTN, hypertension; BP, blood pressure.

The history should assess the duration and severity of hypertension and the presence of risk factors, including a family history. The responses contribute to calculating overall cardiovascular risk.

A full cardiovascular examination includes:
- Blood pressure measurement
- Assessing for hypertensive complications, including fundoscopy
- Detection of a secondary cause.

Measurement of blood pressure An initial reading of >140/90 mmHg should trigger a repeat measurement; if this differs significantly from the first, a third measurement is taken. The recorded blood pressure is the lower of the latter two readings (see page 120).

ABPM or home blood pressure monitoring (HBPM) are more accurate than in-clinic measurements and should be used, when possible, to confirm a diagnosis of hypertension or inform prognosis. More measurements can easily be taken and they reduce the distortion of 'white coat syndrome', where values are raised by patient anxiety. The choice between ABPM and HBPM is influenced by local policy and resources, but ABPM is simpler and perhaps more representative of what is 'normal' for most patients.

Ambulatory blood pressure monitoring ABPM devices typically record blood pressure every 2 h over 24 h; the average waking blood pressure is used to make decisions about treatment.

> ## Clinical insight
>
> Home blood pressure monitors are increasingly cheap and readily available. Self-measurement also helps engage people in their own management, but patients must receive education and training on their use and interpretation.

Home blood pressure monitoring HBPM recordings are usually taken by the patient using a semi-automated device at rest, in a seated position, several times daily over 5–7 days. Measurements are recorded in a blood pressure diary.

Complications   Chronic hypertension may present with its complications, caused by atherosclerotic ischemic damage to organ systems (**Table 4.4**). Damage can occur in major vessels, such as the aorta, or in arteries or arterioles. Fundoscopy, for example, is the only direct way to assess arterial damage, and may show hypertensive retinopathy (see page 123).

Detection of a secondary cause   Secondary hypertension is more likely in younger patients, resistant to therapy and accompanied by features of a primary disease (see page 198). The commonest causes are renal, vascular, endocrine, and neurological disease and drugs.

Investigations

Laboratory investigations are used to:
- Estimate cardiovascular risk, including assessment of diabetes and hyperlipidemia

Organ system	Complication	Presentation
Cardiac	Left ventricular hypertrophy Diastolic heart failure Arrhythmia (especially atrial fibrillation) Ischemic heart disease	Forcible and displaced apex beat (See chapter 9) Myocardial infarction and angina
Renal	Hypertensive nephropathy Renal insufficiency End-stage renal disease	Deranged kidney function tests
Cerebral	Cerebrovascular accident White matter ischemia Hypertensive encephalopathy (at very high blood pressure)	Symptoms and signs of stroke Impaired cognition or dementia Altered mental state, seizures, tremor, myoclonus, asterixis
Ophthalmic	Hypertensive retinopathy	Loss of visual acuity

Table 4.4 The complications of hypertension and their presentation.

- Assess for evidence of end organ damage in the heart, eyes and kidneys (**Table 4.5**)
- Identify secondary causes, especially in young patients with significantly raised or refractory hypertension (see page 198).

The presence of end organ damage indicates a greater risk of cardiovascular events and death, and such cases need aggressive treatment and monitoring.

Blood tests An elevated fasting blood glucose increases cardiovascular risk, whereas a normal result excludes diabetes. A lipid profile (see page 125) with raised total cholesterol, LDL and triglycerides represents increased cardiovascular risk and may indicate treatment.

Urea and electrolytes are measured as raised urea and creatinine occurs in renal impairment, which can both cause, or be a result of, hypertension.

Urinalysis Proteinuria is detected on dipstick testing or a 24 hour urine collection >150 mg per day. It occurs in renal disease and malignant hypertension.

Electrocardiography LVH may be seen on ECG as tall R waves in chest leads V5 and V6 and correspondingly deep S-waves in leads V1 to V4, reflecting thickened myocardium.

Organ	Investigations	Looking for
Heart	12-lead electrocardiogram	Left ventricular hypertrophy and signs of ischemic heart disease
Kidneys	Laboratory tests • Urea and electrolytes • Creatinine clearance • eGFR	Impaired renal function
Eyes	Dipstick urinalysis	Proteinuria (including microalbuminuria) and hematuria (signs of glomerular damage)
	Fundoscopy	Hypertensive retinopathy

Table 4.5 Investigations to assess for end organ damage in hypertension. eGFR, estimated glomerular filtration rate.

Imaging Cerebrovascular and cardiovascular disease are common in older patients with hypertension. Cerebral computerized tomography (CT) or magnetic resonance imaging (MRI) is used to assess for small vessel ischaemic (white matter) changes or evidence of previous cerebrovascular accidents (CVA) in those with memory problems.

Echocardiography is a more sensitive technique to detect LVH than ECG, and is particularly indicated in younger hypertensives.

Management

The European Society of Hypertension/European Society of Cardiology (ESH/ESC) 2013 guidelines, the UK's National Institute for Health and Care Excellence (NICE) 2011 and the American Heart Association/American College of Cardiology (AHA/ACC) 2007 guidelines all propose a stepped approach to treatment, with targets proportional to the patient's cardiovascular risk score (see pages 145 and 305), blood pressure and evidence of end organ damage (**Figure 4.2**). Those with established IHD, cerebrovascular disease or PVD are automatically classified as high risk and should be considered for secondary prevention of CHD. For others, a 10-year cardiovascular risk >20% is considered significant, and should be considered for primary prevention of CHD.

Encourage all patients with high-normal or high blood pressure to aim for healthy lifestyle targets (**Table 4.6**). Antihypertensives may be considered in patients with high-normal blood pressure with a high cardiovascular risk or evidence of end organ damage.

> ### Clinical insight
>
> Informing patients of their cardiovascular risk reinforces advice regarding lifestyle changes and may improve adherence to drug therapy.

Stage of hypertension Management depends on the stage of hypertension (**Table 4.2**):
- Isolated stage 1 hypertension – patients are first advised to make lifestyle modifications; antihypertensives may be

Risk factor	Target	Rationale
Salt intake	<6 g/day: stop adding to food and avoid processed food	Excessive salt consumption increases blood pressure (see above)
Diet	Diet rich in fruits, vegetables, and reduced in saturated and total fat	Thought to have beneficial effects on the renin–angiotensin–aldosterone system, natriuresis, decresed adrenergic tone, and increased vascular relaxation
Weight	BMI <25 kg/m²	Obesity predisposes to hypertension (see above)
Exercise	30 min or more of aerobic exercise on most days of the week	A sedentary lifestyle predispose people to hypertension and atherosclerosis
Alcohol intake	Men <3 or 4 units (24–32 g) and women <2 or 3 units (16–24 g) per day	Alcohol consumption correlates with blood pressure Excessive consumption may antagonize pharmacological treatment
Smoking	Stop	Smoking is a major risk factor for hypertension, IHD and stroke

Table 4.6 Targets for reducing blood pressure by lifestyle modifications. BMI, body mass index.

necessary if the response to these changes is suboptimal
- Stage 1 hypertension with increased cardiovascular risk or end organ damage, as well as those with stage 2 or 3 hypertension, require antihypertensives and lifestyle modification
- Stage 3 hypertension – drug therapy is started immediately, before further diagnostic testing, risk calculation or evidence of end organ damage.

Elderly patients Although blood pressure increases with age as arteries naturally stiffen, treating hypertension is still effective, even in patients over 80 years of age.

Elderly patients taking antihypertensives require close monitoring for adverse effects, contraindications and polypharmacy-related interactions. Postural hypotension is common and can cause falls and reduced mobility.

Patients with diabetes mellitus   Hypertensive patients with diabetes mellitus are at additional risk of cardiovascular disease, retinopathy, renal damage and peripheral neuropathy, and the target blood pressure should be <130/80 mmHg. This is often difficult to achieve, but the benefits of control are greater than in non-diabetic patients.

Patients with coexisting diseases   Antihypertensive drug choice is influenced by the presence of coexisting diseases, due to contraindications or a combined benefit. Preferred drugs include:

- IHD: beta-blockers, angiotensin-converting enzyme (ACE) inhibitors and angiotensin II receptor blockers (ARBs)
- Heart failure: ACE inhibitors, ARBs and potassium-sparing diuretics such as spironolactone
- Renal impairment: antagonists of the renin–angiotensin system (ACE inhibitors and ARBs) reduce blood pressure and proteinuria.

Pregnant patients   More than 10% of pregnant women experience hypertension during pregnancy, including new onset or exacerbation of existing chronic hypertension. It occurs due to hormonal and circulatory changes, but may also indicate placental dysfunction.

Although usually benign, hypertension during pregnancy increases the risk of potentially fatal preeclampsia and eclampsia, and requires specialist management.

Clinical insight

Metabolic syndrome is the association of at least three of:

- Central obesity – the key feature
- Insulin resistance (i.e. type 2 diabetes mellitus)
- Hypertension
- Dyslipidemia – high serum triglycerides, and low high-density lipoproteins (HDLs)

It is a powerful risk factor for cardiovascular disease and death and is increasing significantly, with 25–30% of US and western European adults affected. There is a genetic predisposition but the main causes appear to be a poor and excessive diet and a sedentary lifestyle.

Preeclampsia presents with worsening hypertension and proteinuria during pregnancy and can lead to seizures in late pregnancy: eclampsia.

Antihypertensive drug therapy is limited by fetal side effects, but options include beta-blockers (e.g. labetalol), methyldopa and hydralazine.

Lifestyle changes All patients with hypertension require counseling about how and why to modify their cardiovascular risk (**Table 4.6**). This includes calculation and clear discussion of their overall cardiovascular risk. Referral may be useful for dietary advice, physical training or specialist smoking cessation services in patients that struggle to make positive changes without additional support.

Lifestyle changes may have other benefits, including increased general fitness and energy, improved self-esteem and can decrease the risk of other diseases such as lung cancer, colon cancer, and alcohol dependence.

Medication (Figure 4.3)

Antihypertensive drugs (see page 159) include:
- ACE inhibitors and ARBs
- Beta-blockers

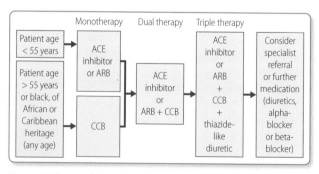

Figure 4.3 Pharmacological treatment of essential hypertension. ACE, angiotensin-converting enzyme; ARB, angiotensin II receptor blocker; CCB, calcium channel blocker.

- Calcium channel blockers
- Diuretics, chiefly thiazide and thiazide-like diuretics
- Alpha-blockers.

The ESH/ESC 2013, NICE 2011 and the AHA/ACC 2007 guidelines all advise a step-wise approach for escalating medication to reach BP targets (**Figure 4.3**):

1. Step 1: monotherapy
2. Step 2: dual therapy
3. Step 3: triple therapy.

> ## Clinical insight
>
> Hypertension is more common in people of African descent, who tend to have low-renin, salt-sensitive hypertension that is less responsive to ACE inhibitor, ARB or beta-blocker monotherapy.

Many patients require dual therapy. Drug choice when considering a third medication is very case-dependent, and diet and lifestyle factors should still be considered. If three drugs do not work, patient adherence should be assessed. If non-adherence is identified, improved patient education is required, with clear instructions on treatment regimen.

4. Step 4: if adherence is not a problem, the patient is considered to have resistant hypertension, indicating assessment for secondary causes (see page 198), specialist referral and/or adding, for example:

- Spironolactone, another diuretic, alpha-blocker or beta blocker (NICE 2011)
- A long-acting thiazide diuretic (e.g. chlorthalidone), spironolactone or the diuretic amiloride (AHA 2008)
- An aldosterone-blocking diuretic (e.g. spironolactone), amiloride and/or the alpha-blocker doxazocin (ESH/ESC 2013).

The primary goal is tight control of blood pressure to prevent atherosclerosis. Drug regimen guidelines vary but drug choice is determined by:

- Effects on blood pressure
- Ethnicity
- Age
- Coexisting diseases
- Previous adverse effects
- Cost-effectiveness.

ACE inhibitors and ARBs are ideal first-line drugs for patients with both hypertension and diabetes as they protect against the nephropathy that both diseases can cause. However, they are not first-line in elderly and African-Caribbean patients who often have low-renin hypertension, but can be used in combination with a diuretic or a calcium channel blocker in these patients as part of dual or triple therapy (see **Figure 4.3**).

Monitoring blood pressure targets Blood pressure should be monitored regularly to achieve treatment targets of:

- <140/90 mmHg in individuals under 80 years
- <150/85 mmHg in those over 80 years
- <130/80 mmHg in patients with diabetes, high cardiovascular risk or renal dysfunction.

Pressures should ideally be measured at least every 5 years in those with normal BP measurements.

Prognosis The degree of end organ damage and the level of cardiovascular risk determine prognosis. Every 20/10 mmHg increase in blood pressure doubles the risk of cardiovascular mortality.

4.3 Secondary hypertension

In approximately 5% of patients with hypertension, it occurs secondary to a specific underlying condition, such as renal artery stenosis (**Figure 4.4** and **Table 4.7**).

Clinical features

Secondary hypertension is usually differentiated from essential hypertension by the presence of features of the underlying disease (**Table 4.7**). Patients are usually under 40 and present with:

- Unexpectedly severe hypertension
- Refractory hypertension

Figure 4.4 Renal artery stenosis. (a) Magnetic resonance angiogram showing left renal artery stenosis ① and post-stenosis dilatation ②. (b) Invasive angiogram showing multiple stenoses in the left renal artery ①. The dark tube in the descending aorta is the catheter, which is injecting contrast dye (black) into the artery.

- Irregular features, such as weakness or profuse sweating
- Proteinuria or hematuria, suggesting renal disease
- Hypokalemia not caused by diuretic use.

Investigations

Investigations for a secondary cause are indicated based on on clinical suspicion, on an individual, case-by-case basis. If a secondary cause is suspected but the cause remains unknown, a good general investigative work-up is outlined in **Table 4.8**.

Management

The underlying cause needs to be treated, and this may involve medication, surgery or even renal dialysis. Antihypertensive medication may also be required while the cause is being corrected; this may need to continue if blood pressure does not normalize.

Prognosis Prognosis is determined by the underlying cause. Prompt diagnosis and treatment that successfully decreases the blood pressure indicates a good prognosis.

Disease	Further information	Investigations
Chronic kidney disease	Commonest cause of secondary HTN	Creatinine clearance or estimated GFR
Polycystic kidney disease	Causes severe resistant HTN Often autosomal dominant hereditability	Renal ultrasound Kidneys may be palpable
Renal artery stenosis	Causes resistant HTN Usually due to atherosclerosis	Renal Doppler ultrasound, CT or MRI angiography
Pheochromocytoma	Very rare cause of severe HTN A catecholamine-secreting tumor	(24-h urinary collection) Catecholamines or their metabolites CT or MRI to identify tumor
Primary hyperaldosteronism	Causes HTN associated with hypokalemia Most commonly due to aldosterone-secreting adenoma (Conn's syndrome)	Plasma K^+ Aldosterone–renin ratio (increased) CT or MRI to identify tumor
Cushing's syndrome	Caused by excessive exposure to corticosteroids or Cushing's disease – (due to ACTH-secreting pituitary tumor)	Cortisol (24-h urine collection) Dexamethasone suppression test CT or MRI to identify tumor
Aortic coarctation	Causes HTN due to congenital narrowing of aorta (usually close to the arch)	Echocardiogram or CT scan
Hormone replacement therapy, oral contraceptives, corticosteroids, NSAIDs, mineralocorticoids	Drug history is very important in hypertension	Drug history

Table 4.7 *Continued...*

Disease	Further information	Investigations
Alcohol, nicotine or liquorice excess; drug misuse	Excessive use is associated with HTN	
Obstructive sleep apnea	Increasingly common cause of HTN associated with obesity. Morning headaches are common	Overnight sleep studies (oximetry and polysomnography) Collateral history from partner is useful
Pregnancy	HTN occurs in 10% of pregnancies	

Table 4.7 Causes of secondary hypertension (HTN). ACTH, adrenocorticotropic hormone; GFR, glomerular filtration rate

Type	Tests	Disease
Examination	Body mass index Radiofemoral delay Abdominal bruit	Obesity Aortic coarctation Renal artery stenosis
Blood tests	Estimated glomerular filtration rate Parathyroid hormone Thyroid-stimulating hormone Calcium Potassium Aldosterone–renin ratio	Renal impairment Hyperparathyroidism Hyperthyroidism Hypercalcemia (sometimes secondary to renal insufficiency) Hypokalemia in aldosteronism Aldosteronism
24-h urine	Cortisol Catecholamines Metanephrines	Cushing's syndrome Pheochromocytoma Pheochromocytoma
Imaging	Renal ultrasound (including Doppler)	Renal artery stenosis, polycystic kidney disease
Others	Sleep studies (if obese or history suggests obstructive sleep apnea)	Obstructive sleep apnea

Table 4.8 Investigations for secondary hypertension.

4.4 Hypertensive emergencies

Hypertensive emergencies are conditions that present with severe uncontrolled hypertension leading to end organ damage. They include accelerated hypertension and hypertension associated with:

- Encephalopathy (usually >200/110 mmHg)
- LVF
- Myocardial ischemia or infarction
- Aortic dissection
- Cerebral hemorrhage
- Acute kidney injury (e.g. glomerulonephritis)
- Pheochromocytoma.

> **Clinical insight**
>
> Rapid decreases in blood pressure should be avoided due to the risk of underperfusion of tissues, particularly the cerebrum.

Hypertensive emergencies can present with cerebral or pulmonary edema, seizures, heart or renal failure. Urgent blood pressure reduction with close supervision is required in a secondary care setting. Intravenous glyceryl trinitrate or labetalol are used to reduce blood pressure above >220/120 mmHg or if there is dangerous secondary pathology.

The aim is to bring systolic blood pressure below 220 mmHg or diastolic blood pressure below 120 mmHg (or both) over 1–2 h, and then <160/100 mmHg over the next 12–24 h.

Hyperlipidemia

Hyperlipidemia is chronic raised blood concentration of tri-glycerides (TG), cholesterol or lipoprotein. It is common but usually subclinical and discovered in screening blood tests of cardiovascular risk assessment.

It has inherited causes, including familial hypercholesterol-emia, and acquired causes such as diet and smoking.

Most types of hyperlipidemia increase the risk and rate of atherogenesis, the deposition of lipid-laden macrophages in arterial walls. It is an important, but often readily treatable, risk factor for coronary heart disease (CHD). A recent study suggests 45% of myocardial infarctions are associated with hyperlipidemia.

Lipid metabolism involves transport lipoproteins that are pro- and anti-atherogenic (see page 68). Hypertriglyceridemia is not directly atherogenic but is associated with remnant lipo-protein particles that are.

5.1 Clinical scenario

Skin lesions and chest pain

Presentation

Bill Hansen, a 42-year-old man, presents to his primary care doctor concerned about chest pain and yellow 'blotches' that have appeared on his ankles and posterior hand in the last few months. He smokes 20 cigarettes a day. He appears concerned but otherwise well, and has BMI of 25.

Diagnostic approach

His chest pain must be characterized and his cardiovascular risk factors should be assessed.

Nodular lesions on the dorsal hand could be warts, abrasions secondary to trauma or xanthomas – cutaneous deposits of foam cells and indicators of hyperlipidemia.

Clinical insight

Xanthomata lipid deposits occur in skin, e.g. as xantholesma, when blood concentrations are high as the skin is an active site of lipid metabolism.

Further history

Bill's chest pain is central, occurs on significant exertion and radiates to his left shoulder and elbow.

Bill's father had a fatal heart attack at the age of 48, and his grandfather died of a stroke at the age of 53.

Diagnostic approach

Bill's chest pain appears anginal, indicating blood tests including a CBC, U&Es, TFTs and LFTs, and an ECG and an exercise stress test. Troponoin levels are only measured if he has had chest pain within the preceding 24 hours.

His family history indicates that he may be at risk from early cardiovascular disease.

Examination

Cardiovascular examination reveals xanthoma tendinosum of the metacarpal and Achilles tendons, xanthelasma around the eyes, and tar-stained fingers. Auscultation reveals a left-sided carotid bruit. His peripheries are cold and no dorsalis pedis pulse can be detected in his left foot.

Diagnostic approach

Xanthomas are cholesterol deposits. Their presence often signals consistently excessive blood cholesterol levels. The carotid bruit likely reflects atherosclerotic narrowing and needs urgent assessment with duplex ultrasound to assess its extent and the risk of cerebrovascular accident. His absent dorsalis pedis pulses and cold feet likely indicate peripheral vascular disease due to femoral or iliac atherosclerosis.

With evidence of hyperlipidemia and atherosclerosis, he has a high risk of cardiovascular disease. He is therefore referred to a cardiologist for electrocardiogram (ECG), exercise stress test and blood tests to assess all cardiovascular risk factors.

Investigations

ECG is normal. Exercise stress testing is positive, indicating probable coronary artery disease. His blood test results are given in **Table 5.1**.

Diagnosis

His angina and investigations suggest Bill already has coronary artery disease, and he is at very high risk of the clinical sequelae of this condition. His blood tests show very high total cholesterol and LDL levels that are unlikely to be due to a secondary cause (e.g. diabetes, liver, renal or thyroid disease).

Bill is diagnosed with definite heterozygous familial hypercholesterolemia according to the Simon Broome criteria (see page 220). This an autosomal dominant inherited hyperlipidaemia due to mutations in LDL receptor genes.

He is counseled about lifestyle and diet changes to lower his total cholesterol and is also started on statins. He is also referred for genetic counseling to inform him of the inherited nature of the disease and ramifications of the diagnosis.

Blood test	Value
Total cholesterol	9.6 mmol/L (370 mg/dL) – *raised*
LDL cholesterol	7.1 mmol/l (275 mg/dL) – *raised*
Triglycerides	3.5 mmol/L (310 mg/dL)
HDL cholesterol	0.8 mmol/L (30 mg/dL)
Glucose (non-fasting)	8.3 mmol/L (150 mg/dL)
Alanine aminotransferase	55 IU/L
Aspartate aminotransferase	65 IU/L
TSH	3.56 mIU/L

Table 5.1 Bill's blood test results. LDL, low-density lipoprotein; HDL, high-density lipoprotein; BUN, blood urea nitrogen; TSH, thyroid-stimulating hormone.

> ## Clinical insight
>
> The World Health Organization (WHO) estimated in 2002 that 60% of CHD in developed countries is attributable to a cholesterol level >3.8 mmol/L (146.7 mg/dL)

At 8-week follow up, his total cholesterol has decreased to 6.4 mmol/L (250 mg/dL). He requires monitoring every 6 months for fasting lipid tests and clinical assessment and may need intervention for his carotid and coronary artery disease. With his relatively early intervention, his prognosis will be much improved but only if he maintains good control of his risk factors and stops smoking.

5.2 Hyperlipidemia

Hyperlipidemia is a significantly raised blood concentration of total cholesterol (e.g. >6.5 mmol/L or 240 mg/dL), lipoprotein or TG. Most forms are associated with an increased risk of atherosclerosis. It can be primary, with no identifiable cause, or it can occur secondary to diabetes mellitus, obesity, pancreatitis or renal disease.

Raised LDL is associated with increased atherogenesis, whereas raised high-density lipoprotein (HDL) is protective, as the former increases arterial wall lipid deposition and macrophage accumulation, and the latter decreases it.

Types

Types of hyperlipidemia include:
- Hypercholesterolemia – raised cholesterol
- Hypertriglyceridemia – raised TG
- Chylomicronemia – raised chylomicrons
- Dysbetalipoproteinemia – raised intermediate density lipoproteins (IDLs) and TG and lowered HDL
- Mixed hyperlipoproteinemia, raised VLDL and chylomicrons
- Combined hyperlipoproteinemia – rasied chylomicrons and TG.

Primary hyperlipidemias are distinguished by the Fredrickson classification, based on separation of blood lipids by centrifuge or electrophoresis. Primary forms usually present with extreme lipid levels, family history and xanthoma, and patients should be referred to a specialist lipid clinic.

An increase in chylomicrons or VLDL leads to an increase in TG. An increase in LDL or IDL causes an increase in cholesterol.

Clinical insight

Dyslipidemia refers to abnormal levels of lipids in the blood, including low levels of HDLs. Hyperlipidemia is the most common dyslipidemia, and is usually due to a high fat diet and sedentary lifestyle.

Epidemiology

Nearly 31 million US adults have hyperlipidemia with a total cholesterol ≥240 mg/dL (≥6.2 mmol/L). It is closely associated with a Westernized diet and lifestyle. It is more common in men. Total and LDL cholesterol rises 20% from the age of 20 to 50 years.

Primary inherited hyperlipidemias include familial combined hyperlipidemia (FCH) and familial hypertriglyceridemia, two of the most prevalent genetic disorders (**Table 5.2**). FCH is implicated in 10% of CHD patients.

Etiology

Lipids are transported as lipoproteins, of which there are five types based on size and density (see page 80):

- Chylomicrons carry lipids from the intestine to the liver, muscle and adipose tissue
- VLDLs carry TGs from liver to adipose tissue
- IDLs are not usually detectable
- LDLs carry lipid around the body
- HDLs collect peripheral lipid and take it to the liver.

Size is important as this reflects a lipoprotein's role in metabolism and therefore disease. As metabolic pathways interconnect lipoproteins, the amount of one type is affected by the concentration of others. Each is associated with a different level of atherogenesis (i.e. cardiovascular risk). For example, raised LDL is associated with an increased risk, a high level of chylomicrons is not associated with increased risk, and HDL actually decreases cardiovascular risk.

Type	Raised elements	Example	Approximate prevalence
I	Cholesterol, TG, chylomicrons	Familial hyperchylomicronemia (decreased lipoprotein lipase or apolipoprotein (apo) CII)	1/1,000,000
IIa	Cholesterol, LDL	Familial hypercholesterolemia (loss of LDL receptors, see page 217)	Homozygous – 1/1,000,000 Heterozygous – 1/500
IIb	Cholesterol, TG, LDL, VLDL	Familial combined hypercholesterolemia	1/200
III	Cholesterol, TG, IDL	Familial dysbetalipoproteinemia (apo E2 mutation) causing impaired VLDL clearance	1/10,000
IV	TG, VLDL	Familial hypertriglyceridemia (increased VLDL synthesis or decreased breakdown)	1/100
V	Cholesterol, TG, VLDL, chylomicrons	Familial combined hyperlipidemia (loss of lipoprotein lipase; increased VLDL synthesis)	1/50 – 1/200

Table 5.2 The Fredrickson classification of primary hyperlipoproteinemias. TG, triglyceride; IDL, intermediate-density lipoprotein; LDL, low-density lipoprotein; VLDL, very low-density lipoprotein; apo E2, apolipoprotein E2.

Moderate or severely raised TG levels are substantial risk factors for cardiovascular disease and long term mortality, although the high levels of Type I hyperlipidemia are, surprisingly, not associated with increased atherogenesis.

Primary

Primary causes are genetic (see **Table 5.2**) or idiopathic.

System	Disease	Pathophysiology	Lipid profile
Endocrine disorders	Diabetes mellitus	Increased production and reduced removal of TG	↑ TG ↓ HDL
	Hypothyroidism	Decreased LDL receptor activity	↑ LDL, TC ↓ normal TG
Renal disorders	Nephrotic syndrome	Increased LDL production, reduced VLDL clearance	↑ TC, LDL. ↑ normal TG
	Renal failure	Impaired TG breakdown	↑ LDL, TG. ↓ HDL
Drugs	Adrenal steroids	Increased hepatic fatty acid synthesis	↑ LDL and HDL
	Thiazides	Likely due to decreased insulin sensitivty and/or reflex RAAS and SNS activation	↑ TC, LDL, TG
	Anticonvulsants	Likely via hepatic enzyme induction and increased cholesterol absorption	Raised TC, TG, HDL
	Oral contraceptives	Increased hepatic VLDL production	↑ LDL, HDL and TG
	Alcohol	Inhibits chylomicron breakdown	↑ TG, HDL
Hepatic disease	Obstructive liver disease	Reduced hepatic lipoprotein metabolsm	↑ Free cholesterol, LDL ↑normal HDL
	Hepatitis		↑ TG, LDL ↑ TC, HDL

Table 5.3 *Continued...*

System	Disease	Pathophysiology	Lipid profile
Storage diseases	Gaucher disease	Liver malfunction due to glucocerebroside accumulation	↓ HDL
	Von Gierke disease	Low insulin causes hypertriglyceridemia	↑ TG ↑ normal TC
	Systemic lupus erythematosus	Low HDL	↑ normal TC, LDL, TG ↓ HDL
Other	Obesity	Increased free fatty acids to liver reduces apoB breakdown, increases TG release by lipoproteins	↑ TG ↑ normal TC, LDL

Table 5.3 Causes of secondary hyperlipidemia. TG, triglyceride; LDL, low density lipoprotein; VLDL, very low density lipoprotein; apoB, apolipoprotein B.

Secondary causes

Hyperlipidemia can occur due to other causes including systemic disease or drugs (**Table 5.3**). The most common cause is poor diet and a sedentary lifestyle, which may be associated with metabolic syndrome including diabetes mellitus type II.

> ## Guiding principle
>
> All cells can make cholesterol, but liver cells are the most active. It is also consumed in the diet, particularly egg yolk, cheese, butter, liver, oily fish, and many processed foods.

There is a normal increase in blood lipid concentrations following a meal – postprandial hyperlipidemia. A high fat, low fiber diet leads to increased circulating lipoproteins and TGs and a sedentary lifestyle means that levels stay raised for longer.

Clinical features

Most patients are asymptomatic and hyperlipidemia is diagnosed by blood tests. Xanthomas may be present in patients with very high lipid levels, usually indicating an inherited cause. These are sub-cutaneous usually raised, yellow-orange or reddish-brown deposits of lipid–laden foam cells. They can be solitary or 'eruptive' collections:

- Xanthelasma around the eyes or on the eyelids, the most common form (**Figure 5.1**)

Figure 5.1 Xanthelasma. Yellowish papules and plaques of lipid-laden foam cells in xanthelasma palpebra.

- Xanthoma planum is a flat deposit; this type of xanthoma occurs at various sites
- Xanthoma tuberosum on the elbows and knees
- Xanthoma tendinosum in tendons (e.g. Achilles' tendon); these xanthomas move with extension and occur later than other xanthomas.

Deposits also occur in the stratum of the cornea, seen as a corneal arcus of gray-white rings.

Associated signs of atherosclerotic disease or hyperlipidemic complications may be present (**Table 5.4**).

Diagnostic approach

Investigation and management of dyslipidemias is always considered in the context of total cardiovascular risk (see page 305). Primary prevention begins by identifying people likely to be at increased risk and performing a full formal risk assessment.

Inherited and secondary causes must be ruled out. Management then focuses on reaching optimal levels or treatment targets, largely of LDL or non-HDL cholesterol, proportional to

System	Clinical feature	Pathogenesis
Cardiovascular	Decreased peripheral pulses or ankle/brachial index	PVD
Respiratory	Dyspnea	CHD, congestive heart failure
Neurologic	Dementia and depression	Chylomicronemia syndrome
Dermatologic	Xanthoma	Deposits of lipid-laden macrophages
Ophthalmologic	Corneal arcus	Esterified cholesterol deposits
Gastrointestinal	Upper right abdominal tenderness Hepatomegaly	Liver disease

Table 5.4 Clinical features associated with hyperlipidemia and associated atherosclerosis. PVD, peripheral vascular disease; CHD, coronary heart disease.

the patient's individual total cardiovascular risk. There is large overlap in international guidelines, for example:

- The American Heart Association and American College of Cardiology (AHA/ACC) (2013)
- The European Society of Cardiology/European Atherosclerosis Society (ESC/EAS) (2011)
- The National Institute for Health and Care Excellence guidelines (NICE) (2014; see **Figure 5.2**).

Once identified at risk, an initial lipid profile is taken. Secondary causes and familial hypercholesterolemia must be considered and tested for before therapy commences for primary prevention of CHD. Suspect familial hypercholesterolemia in a patient with a family history of early CHD, xanthoma and a total cholesterol >7.5 mmol/L (>290 mg/dL).

> ## Clinical insight
>
> Non-fasting blood lipid measurements slightly overestimate CHD risk with a higher TG and lower HDL concentrations. However, the NICE 2014 guidelines consider them sufficient for screening and convenient for patients.

Investigations

Blood tests to specifically investigate dyslipidemia include:

- Full lipid profile – total cholesterol, HDL, non-HDL and TG. According to the NICE 2014 guidelines, this can be a non-fasting sample although a fasting sample is always preferred
- HbA1c to assess for diabetes
- Thyroid stimulating hormone (TSH) level
- U&Es to assess kidney function
- Liver function tests.

Specialist referral is indicated by:

- Total cholesterol >9.0 mmol/L (350 mg/dL)
- Non-HDL >7.5 mmol/L (290 mg/dL).

Management

All recent guidelines recommend key management principles:

- Consider absolute total cardiovascular risk of patient when initiating and monitoring treatment

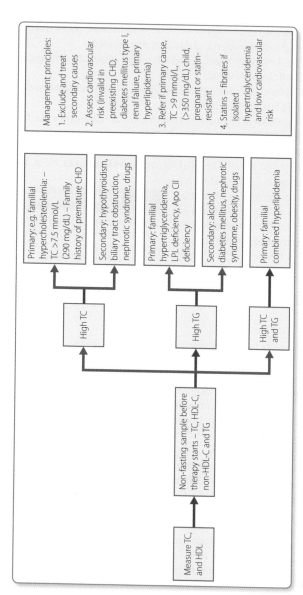

Figure 5.2 Investigation and management principles of hyperlipidemia, based on the UK's NICE 2014 guidelines. TC, total cholesterol; HDL, high-density lipoprotein; TG, triglyceride; CHD, coronary heart disease; LPL, lipoprotein lipase; apo, apolipoprotein.

Patient risk	Criteria		Optimal LDL
	Risk factors	CHD 10-year risk (%)	
High risk	1. Known CHD 2. CHD risk equivalents: a. PVD b. Cerebrovascular disease c. Abdominal aortic aneurysm d. Diabetes mellitus e. 2+ risk factors	>20	<1.8 mmol/L (<70 mg/dL) or a ≥50% reduction from baseline
Moderately high risk	2+ risk factors with CHD	10–20	<2.5 mmol/L (<97 mg/dL)
Moderate risk	2+ risk factors with CHD	<10	<3.0 mmol/L (<116 mg/dL)
Low risk	0–1 risk factors with CHD	<10	<3.0 mmol/L (<116 mg/dL)

Table 5.5 Optimal lipoprotein levels according to overall cardiovascular risk. Based on ESC/EAS 2011 guidelines. Local risk assessment tools and guidelines should be used. Risk factors: smoking, hypertension (≥140/90), HDL <1.0 mmol/L (<40 mg/dL), age ≥45 years (men), >55 years (women), IHD in first-degree relative (<55 years [men], < 65 years [women]). CHD, coronary heart disease; PVD, peripheral vascular disease; LDL, low-density lipoprotein; HDL, high-density lipoprotein.

- Correlate therapeutic intensity with risk level category
- Continue lifestyle and diet recommendations
- Focus on achieving optimal levels of LDL and non-HDL (**Table 5.5**)
- Use statins as first-line therapy if lifestyle modifications are insufficient, or without delay in secondary prevention
- Address issues of adherence including clear communication and managing effective behavioral change.

More recent guidelines do not recommend specific target levels of lipoproteins for the primary or secondary prevention of atherosclerotic disease.

As the main reason for treatment is to decrease cardiovascular risk, hyperlipidaemia is managed in context of total cardiovascular risk (see page 305, **Table 5.5**). Standard risk assessment tools are not valid for those with inherited hyperlipidaemias or other causes of high cardiovascular risk.

The inherited lipidemias respond best to different treatments (**Table 5.6**).

Secondary hyperlipidemia management must focus on treating the underlying cause, where possible. Lipid-lowering medication may also be needed. For example, patients with hypothyroidism should have their thyroid biochemistry corrected before starting lipid-lowering medication. Normalization of thyroid function may be enough to treat the lipid abnormality.

Diet and exercise

Initial treatment is lifestyle modifications including (see page 146):

- Weight loss and exercise
- A diet with restricted saturated fat, trans fats and cholesterol (**Table 5.7**) and modest portion sizes
- Smoking cessation
- Limited alcohol intake.

Lipids are measured again after 3–6 months. If LDL is still raised, medication is considered.

Medication

Medications include (see page 148) 3-hydroxy-3-methyl-glutaryl-CoA (HMG-CoA) reductase inhibitors (statins), the

Type of primary hyperlipidemia	Principal treatment
I	Diet
IIa	Diet, bile acid sequestrants, statins, niacin
IIb	Diet, statins, niacin, fibrate
III	Fibrate, statins
IV	Fibrate, niacin, statins
V	Niacin, fibrate

Table 5.6 Principle treatments for the inherited hyperlipidemias.

Component	Examples	Frequency
Lean protein	Chicken breast, tofu	Every meal
High fiber, low GI carbohydrate	Vegetables, pulses, whole grains, fruits	Every meal
Nuts	Handful	Daily
Leafy greens	Cabbage, spinach	Daily
Highly processed foods	Processed sugar, high fructose corn syrup, trans fats, white flour	Avoid

Table 5.7 A recommended diet to lower blood triglyceride levels.

routine first line medication for primary and secondary prevention of CHD.

Non-statins are not recommended unless the patient is confirmed as intolerant to statins, statin therapy is ineffective or an inherited hyperlipidemia is confirmed (**Table 5.6**):

- Fibrates – particularly useful to lower TG
- Bile acid sequestrants
- Niacin
- Omega 3 fatty acids – as fish oil supplements or purified forms as an adjunct to lifestyle changes.

Lipid levels should be checked 8 weeks after starting or changing medication, until they are satisfactory. Once optimum levels have been achieved, lipids are checked annually.

Clinical insight

Statin side effects include:

- Elevated liver function tests
- Myopathy – evident as Increased muscle creatine phosphokinase (CPK)
- Rhabdomyolysis (rare) – secondary to myopathy.

If a patient's CPK level is ≥5 times normal, stop treatment, check renal function, and monitor every 2 weeks.

5.3 Familial hypercholesterolemia

Familial hypercholesterolemia (FH) is an autosomal dominant condition that leads to extreme levels of LDL but normal TG. This increases the incidence of premature atherosclerosis and CHD. However, the risk is dramatically reduced if the condition is identified and treated. It is one of the most common inherited conditions.

Epidemiology and etiology

Many different mutations have been identified. Most affect the *LDLR* gene on chromosome 19, which encodes the LDL receptor. Mutations lead to absent or significantly dysfunctioning LDL receptors (**Figure 5.3**).

Homozygous FH

Homozygotes have a mutation in both copies of *LDLR*, which leads to a more serious condition and a life expectancy under 30 years, if untreated. It affects one in a million people, and presents in childhood with signs of atherosclerosis.

Heterozygous FH

1 in 250/500 people have heterozygous familial hypercholesterolemia, with a single mutant *LDLR* gene. Untreated, about 50% of men and 30% of women have clinical CHD by the age

Figure 5.3 Familial hypercholesterolemia most often involves dysfunctioning mutations of low-density lipoprotein (LDL) receptors. Intermediate-density lipoproteins (IDLs) are not taken up via LDL receptors on the liver, leading to increased LDL formation. apo, apolipoprotein; CE, cholesteryl ester; CETP, cholesteryl ester transfer protein; CHOL, cholesterol; FFA, free fatty acids; HDL, high-density lipoprotein; TG, triglycerides; VLDL, very low-density lipoprotein.

of 50. The majority remain undiagnosed until a cardiovascular event.

Clinical features

Features of cutaneous or vascular lipid deposits are earlier and more severe in homozygous disease.

Homozygous FH

Homozygotes present with signs of atherosclerosis in childhood: features of aortic stenosis, peripheral vascular or cerebrovascular disease, or, particularly, CHD. Nearly all homozygotes develop xanthoma (see page 119), initially as dispersed flat lesions and evolving to xanthoma tendinosum and xanthelasma by the early childhood.

Heterozygous FH

Heterozygote children do not usually have signs, but will likely have a parent with severe hypercholesteremia and a family history of cardiovascular disease.

Adults may present with:

- Long history of severe hypercholesterolemia
- Angina or myocardial infarction, peripheral vascular or cerebrovascular disease.
- 60% of those over 20 who are untreated have xanthoma tendinosum on the Achilles or metacarpal extensor tendons
- Xanthelasma (**Figure 5.1**).

> **Clinical insight**
>
> Homozygous familial hypercholesterolemia is associated with severe atherosclerosis in carotid, coronary, femoral and iliac arteries, highlighting the metabolic component of this inflammatory-metabolic disease. Patients have a four-fold risk of CHD.

Diagnostic approach

Familial hypercholesterolemia is diagnosed according to the Simon Broome criteria (**Table 5.8**). The diagnosis is either definite or possible, depending on the presence of tendon xanthomas, family history of myocardial infarction, and serum cholesterol concentrations.

It is estimated that up to 90% of patients with FH are undiagnosed. Early recognition and treatment can vastly improve outcome.

Adult TC > 7.5 mmol/L (290 mg/dL) or LDL > 4.9 mmol/L (200 mg/dL) OR Child (age < 16 years) TC > 6.7 mmol/L (260 mg/dL) or LDL > 4 mmol/L (155 mg/dL)	
And	
Xanthoma tendinosum in the patient, or a first- or second-degree relative Or DNA evidence of a known mutation associated with family history	Family history of myocardial infarction (< 60 years in a first-degree relative; < 50 years in a second-degree relative) Or Family history of increased total cholesterol > 7.5 mmol/L (290 mg/dL) in a first- or second-degree adult relative; > 6.7 mmol/L (260 mg/dL) in a child or sibling younger than 16 years)
↓ **Definite FH**	↓ **Possible FH**

Table 5.8 The Simon Broome criteria for the diagnosis of familial hypercholesterolemia (FH). These are initial, fasting tests. TC, total cholesterol; LDL, low-density lipoprotein.

Management

Patients are referred to a specialist lipid clinic. The target reduction in serum total cholesterol and LDL cholesterol is 50% of baseline values. All patients require lifestyle modifications, including:

- Smoking cessation
- Weight loss and exercise
- A diet with restricted saturated fat, trans fats and cholesterol.

Homozygotes require intense lipid-lowering therapy with statins as first-line therapy. If lipid concentrations remain above the targets, a second agent (usually ezetimibe) is recommended.

Coronary heart disease

Coronary heart disease (CHD) – also known as ischemic heart disease (IHD) or coronary artery disease (CAD) – is a reduction in blood supply to the myocardium, usually caused by atherosclerosis. Less common causes include non-embolic thrombosis, infective emboli, systemic vascular diseases and coronary artery dissection.

CHD is the leading cause of death and serious illness in the developed world, and quickly becoming so in the developing world. In the UK, for example, CHD is responsible for 20% of male and 14% of female deaths. Worldwide it causes 12.8% of all deaths.

Patients can be asymptomatic, or, if demand for oxygen exceeds supply, with central chest pain on exertion (i.e. angina). If an atherosclerotic plaque ruptures and occludes a coronary artery, patients are at risk of acute coronary syndromes (ACS):

- Unstable angina
- Non-ST elevation myocardial infarction (NSTEMI)
- ST elevation myocardial infarction (STEMI).

Therapies focus on controlling risk factors, reducing myocardial oxygen demand, reopening blocked arteries and reducing blood coagulability.

6.1 Clinical scenario

Pain radiating across chest and down left arm

Presentation

Dan Taylor (58 years old) presents to the emergency department complaining of a central chest pain that radiates down his left arm. He has had the pain for 1 week, but it suddenly became worse this morning.

Diagnostic approach

Dan's chest pain should be characterized further, for example using the Socrates mnemonic (Table 2.2) to differentiate the cause (**Table 6.1**).

	Ischemic	Pleuritic	Musculoskeletal
Site	Central, retrosternal	Focal (single finger point)	Variable
Character	Heavy, tight, pressure	Sharp, 'stabbing'	Tender
Precipitating factors	Exercise, cold, heavy meals, stress (anything which increases physical demand on heart)	Deep inspiration and coughing	Movement, postural change, palpation
Relieving factors	Rest and nitrates (if stable angina)	Shallow breathing	Staying still or exertion
Radiation	Into jaw and arms and back	Rare	Rare
Other	Stable angina eases with rest and nitrates – ACS pain does not	Caused by friction between inflamed visceral and parietal pleural/pericardial layers	Tenderness to palpation common

Table 6.1 Characteristics of the main causes of chest pain.

Clinical insight

A 'silent MI' presents with little or no pain, but instead is often dismissed as indigestion, muscle sprain or trapped wind. This is more common in the elderly, diabetics and those with heart transplants.

Further history

Dan's past medical history includes CHD, hypertension, and hypercholesterolemia. He suffers from infrequent angina on exertion, typically resolving with rest or use of glyceryl tri-nitrate (GTN) spray. However, rest or GTN have not worked for the last week. He dismissed the symptoms as indigestion and took an over-the-counter indigestion remedy to no effect. He is not nauseous or dizzy, and has no palpitations.

Diagnostic approach

Episodic pain all week suggests Dan may have unstable angina and a sudden deterioration may be due to a myocardial infarction, although differentials including pulmonary embolism or pericarditis must be excluded.

Patients with a history of angina are usually aware of what their 'normal' pain is. More persistent or severe pain suggests an ACS and immediate medical advice is needed.

Examination

On examination:
- Dan is dyspneic, pale and clammy
- His pulse is 90 bpm
- His blood pressure is 110/60 mmHg
- The JVP is not raised
- The capillary refill time is 2 seconds
- His respiratory rate is 18 per minute
- His oxygen saturation is 95% on room air.

On auscultation, his chest is clear and heart sounds are normal. There is no peripheral edema or fever. His chest pain is not reproducible on palpation and his abdominal examination is unremarkable.

Diagnostic approach

Dan's history suggests his 'usual' angina has become unstable, and may have progressed to MI. Pallor and clamminess due to sympathetic activation are common in patients experiencing severe ischemia and MI.

Investigations

A portable chest X-ray shows clear lung fields; an electrocardiograph (ECG) demonstrates convex ST elevation >5 mm in leads II, III and aVF

Clinical insight

Myocardial infarction often presents with normal examination findings, unless it has caused heart failure or an arrhythmia

(**Figure 6.1**). Baseline blood tests including full blood count, renal function, liver function and troponin are all normal.

Diagnosis

Dan is diagnosed with ST elevation MI (STEMI), as evident on his ECG. ECG also suggests it occurred in the right coronary artery as it is affecting the inferior myocardial territory (**Table 6.2**).

Figure 6.1 Mr Bayliss' electrocardiograph demonstrating convex anterior ST elevation in inferior leads (II, III, aVF) ①, reciprocal changes ②, hyperacute T waves ③ and posterior extension of the infarction ④.

Site of infarct		ST elevation	Culprit vessel
Left ventricle	Anterior	V1–V4	Left anterior descending artery
	Septal	V3–V4	Left anterior descending artery
	Lateral	I, aVL and V5–V6	Left circumflex artery
	Inferior	II, III and avF	Right coronary artery or left circumflex artery
	Posterior	V7–V9	Left circumflex artery
Right ventricle		V1–V2	Right coronary artery

Table 6.2 Localizing infarcts by ECG changes. Note there is significant crossover.

He is transferred to the primary percutaneous coronary intervention (PPCI) center for angioplasty to open the blocked coronary artery.

6.2 Angina

Angina (Gr. *Ankhonē* 'strangling') is chest pain due to myocardial ischemia; the most common presenting symptom of CHD. It is typically described as a 'heavy' or 'crushing' central chest pain on exertion and relieved by rest.

Stable angina only occurs on exertion; unstable angina also occurs at rest. It is graded by its severity and to what degree it limits activity (**Table 6.3**).

Epidemiology

There are over 20,000 new cases of angina a year in the UK. It affects 12% of men and 5% of women over 55 in the UK, and approximately 2% of all adults globally.

Risk factors

Risk factors include those that are modifiable or non-modifiable – important to consider in prevention – and probable factors with unknown mechanisms (**Table 6.4**). The major factors are

Class	Definition
1	Angina only during strenuous or prolonged physical activity
2	Slight limitation, with angina only during vigorous physical activity
3	Symptoms with everyday living activities (i.e. moderate limitation)
4	Inability to perform any activity without angina or angina at rest (i.e. severe limitation)

Table 6.3 The Canadian Cardiovascular Society Angina Grading Scale.

Non-modifiable	Modifiable	Probable
Advanced age	High blood pressure	Obesity
Male gender	Diabetes	Poor diet
Personal history of coronary heart disease	Smoking	Chronic kidney disease
Family history of coronary heart disease	Hypercholesterolemia	

Table 6.4 Modifiable, non-modifiable and probable risk factors for the development of coronary heart disease.

smoking, hypercholesterolemia, hypertension, diabetes and a positive family history: a first-degree relative with premature CHD, i.e. diagnosed before the age of 65 years (**Table 6.5**). Primary prevention focuses on controlling or reversing modifiable risk factors:
• Smoking cessation
• Strict control of hypertension and diabetes
• Regular exercise
• A Mediterranean-style diet, rich in fresh fruit and vegetables.
Calculating the overall cardiovascular risk is an essential part of managing angina and preventing CHD (see pages 145 and 305).

Pathogenesis
Myocardial ischemia can result from:
• Coronary vessel blockage

Type of chest pain	Non-anginal‡				Atypical angina§				Typical angina‖			
Gender	Male		Female		Male		Female		Male		Female	
Degree of risk*,†	Low	High	Low	High	Low	High	Low	High	Low	High	Low	High
Age(years) 35	3	35	1	19	8	59	2	39	30	88	10	78
45	9	47	2	22	21	70	5	43	51	92	20	79
55	23	59	4	25	45	79	10	47	80	95	38	82
65	49	69	9	29	71	86	20	51	93	97	56	84

*Low risk: no diabetes, smoking or hypercholesterolemia.
†High risk: diabetes, smoking or hypercholesterolemia.
‡Non-anginal: one risk factor out of three (diabetes, smoking or hypercholesterolemia) plus constricting discomfort on exertion or improved by rest.
§Atypical anginal: two risk factors out of diabetes, smoking and hypercholesterolemia.
‖Typical anginal: all three risk factors (diabetes, smoking and hypercholesterolemia).

Table 6.5 Percentage likelihood of coronary heart disease, based on symptoms and risk factors. Adapted from National Institute for Health and Care Excellence (NICE). Chest pain of recent onset: assessment and diagnosis of recent onset chest pain or discomfort of suspected cardiac origin. London: NICE; 2013.

- Coronary vessel vasospasm or constriction
- Decreased oxygen in blood.

CHD results from atherosclerotic plaques impinging into the coronary arterial lumen (see page 174) inhibiting blood flow, leading to myocardial anaerobic respiration and compromised function. Angina arises when sensory nerve endings are stimulated mechanically and chemically (e.g. adenosine) in the coronary arteries and myocardium. The nerves travel to the first four thoracic spinal nerves (T1 to T4), the spinal cord, thalamus and then cortex. Pain increases as myocardial metabolic demand does.

> ## Clinical insight
>
> Stable angina is usually precipitated by exertion but quickly resolves (<10 min) with either rest or use of a glyceryl trinitrate spray. ACS is usually more severe, lasts longer and provokes more fear in the patient, or occurs at a lower threshold of exercise or stress.

Clinical features

Chest pain is typically central or retrosternal, and described as crushing or tight; 'like a band across the chest' and may radiate – or be solely localized to – the left arm, arms, the neck or jaw (**Figure 2.1**).

Exacerbating factors include cold, exertion, large meals and stress. Relieving factors include use of glyceryl trinitrate and rest.

Angina is often associated with dyspnea, especially in cases of left ventricular systolic impairment resulting in pulmonary edema.

Clinical signs

Signs of CHD risk factors may be seen:

- Glycosuria or complications of diabetes
- High blood pressure (i.e. hypertension)
- Tar-stained fingers (i.e. smoking)
- Xanthelasma (i.e. hypercholesterolemia)

Investigations

Investigations aim to quickly distinguish angina from non-cardiac chest pain and ACSs. The American Heart Association (AHA)/American College of Cardiology (ACC) 2014 guidelines on the management of patients with Non-ST elevation MI recommend that patients with suspected angina or other ACS symptoms presenting to the emergency department have:

- A 12-lead ECG performed and are evaluated within 10 minutes of arrival
- Troponin I or T blood levels measured at presentation and 3–6 hours post symptom onset
- If no ischemic ECG or biomarker changes are present, non-invasive imaging within 72 hours
- Use of risk scores to guide management and assess prognosis

Less acutely, patients with suspected angina typically undergo ECG at rest, and graded exercise testing if angina is strongly suspected. If present, invasive coronary angiography is performed to investigate CHD severity.

The UK National Institute for Health and Care Excellence (NICE) guidelines help assess the pre-test likelihood of CHD based on the patient's symptoms and risk factors (**Table 6.5**). Similarly, the AHA/ACC 2014 guidelines and European Society of Cardiology (ESC) 2011 guidelines on Non-STEMI management both recommend use of the Global Registry of Acute Coronary Events (GRACE) data for calculating the risk of death or death/MI following an ACS (see www.outcomesumassmed.org/grace/).

Electrocardiography ECG is typically normal in patients with CHD, unless they have had a prior myocardial infarction or there are signs of risk factors such as hypertension. Signs of current ischemia include:

- ST segment depression (**Figure 6.1**)
- T-wave flattening or inversion
- Left bundle branch block.

Functional testing Functional tests use exercise or drugs to precipitate signs of ischemia:

- Exercise ECG
- Single-photon emission computed tomography (SPECT) scanning (also known as perfusion scanning)
- Stress echocardiography
- Magnetic resonance imaging (MRI)

They can help differentiate scarred and ischemic myocardium, and can also indicate the site of the ischemia.

Imaging Coronary anatomy is assessed by coronary computed tomographic angiography (CCTA) and invasive angiography (see pages 142 and 143). CCTA is good at detecting atherosclerotic plaques and calcium in the coronary tree, but invasive angiography is better for assessing disease severity as its higher resolution results in less false positive results. Invasive angiography also allows treatment of the lesion during a single test.

Management

Treatment aims to reduce symptoms, slow CHD progression and reduce the likelihood of future ACS stroke events. Risk factor management for patients diagnosed with stable CHD is summarized in **Table 6.6**.

Medication

Symptomatic therapies reduce cardiac preload and afterload, and increase coronary dilation, by systemic and coronary vasodilation, whereas prognostic therapies improve outcome (**Table 6.7**). The 2012 AHA guidelines on management of stable CHD recommend initial symptomatic therapy of GTN and a beta-blocker, and adding/substituting a calcium channel blocker or long-acting GTN if required.

Surgery

Patients with anginal pain which is unresponsive to medication are considered for percutaneous coronary intervention (PCI), also known as angioplasty (see page 163, Figure 2.31).

Coronary artery bypass graft (CABG) is indicated in patients with severe disease – e.g. affecting all three vessels or with very tight stenosis of the left main stem – or where PCI is unsuitable.

Prognosis

2% of patients with angina will develop ACS every year.

Risk factor	Recommendation
Smoking	Cessation via counselling and/or pharmacology
Blood pressure	Lifestyle modifications (see page 194)
	Target: <160/100 mm Hg (<130/80 in diabetes or CKD)
	Regularly assess blood pressure
	ACE inhibitor* if CV risk is moderate or higher, or in presence of LVEF ≤40%, hypertension, diabetes or CKD
	ARBs for hypertensive patients who are ACEI-intolerant and have HF or a post-MI LVEF ≤40%
	ACE inhibitor/ARB combination therapy for HF due to left ventricular systolic dysfunction
	Aldosterone blockade (e.g. spironolactone) in patients post-MI, with no CKD or hyperkalemia, who have LVEF ≤40%, and diabetes or HF, if hypertension not controlled by ACE inhibitor and beta blocker therapy
	Beta blockers* in patients post-ACS, or with left ventricular dysfunction or HF
Blood lipids	Diet: reduce saturated fat intake (<7% of calorific intake) and trans-fatty acid intake (<1%) and total cholesterol < 5.2 mmol/L (<200 mg/dL)
	Plant sterols (2 g/day) or viscous fiber (10 g/day)
	Omega 3 fatty acids (1 g/day)
	Weight management / physical activity
	Regularly assess fasting lipid profile: • LDL target <1.8 mmol/L (<70 mg/dL) or use high dose statins • If LDL ≥2.6 mmol/L (≥100 mg/dL): start lipid lowering medication and lifestyle modifications or intensify current treatment • High or moderately high risk patients: aim for LDL reduction of 30–40% • If TG 2.3–5.6 mmol/L (200–499 mg/dL), aim for non-HDL <3.4 mmol/L (<130 mg/dL) • If TG ≥2.3 mmol/L (≥200 mg/dL), aim for non-HDL <2.6 mmol/L (<100 mg/dL) After LDL-lowering therapy initiated, niacin or fibrates can lower non-HDL: • If TG ≥5.6 mmol/L (≥500 mg/dL): fibrates or niacin to reduce risk of pancreatitis; aim for non-HDL <3.4 mmol/L (130 mg/dL) Drug combination helps achieve LDL <2.6 mmol/L (<100 mg/dL)

Table 6.6 Summary of risk factor management in patients with chronic stable CHD. Based on the 2012 guidelines from the AHA and others on management of stable CHD. *Continued overleaf*

Risk factor	Recommendation
Physical activity	≤30 minutes 5 times a week Exercise testing to guide exercise prescription Cardiac rehabilitation after recent ACS, revascularization or HF
Weight	Assess regularly: advise BMI maintained at 18.5–24.9 Consider metabolic syndrome treatment strategies if waist >89 cm (35 in) in women, >102 cm (40 in) in men Initial goal: 10% reduction from baseline
Diabetes	Aim for near-normal HbA1c Aggressive treatment of other CV risk factors
Clotting	Aspirin (75–150 mg/day)* Additional anticoagulation with warfarin (requires INR monitoring)

Table 6.6 *Continued.* CKD, chronic kidney disease; ACE, angiotensin-converting enzyme; CV, cardiovascular; LVEF, left ventricular ejection fraction; ARB, angiotensin II receptor blockers; HF, heart failure; MI, myocardial infarction; ACS, acute coronary syndrome; LDL, low-density lipoprotein; HDL; high-density lipoprotein; TG, triglyceride; BMI, body-mass index. *Indefinitely and unless contraindicated.

6.3 Acute coronary syndromes

ACSs are a spectrum of CHD involving severe blockage of the coronary circulation. Like stable angina, they are caused by atherosclerotic deposits in vessel walls preventing sufficient blood flow through the lumen. However, they represent an acute change in the lesion(s) due to plaque rupture, acute thrombosis and/or embolism causing an actual or potential infarction. They all require immediate hospital admission.

Types

There are three main syndromes:

- **Unstable angina:** irregular, significant worsening angina that can occur at rest but with no evidence of infarction; a 'pre-myocardial infarction' condition

Drug group	Mechanism of action	Example
Symptomatic drugs		
Nitrates	NO-induced coronary vasodilation	Glyceryl trinitrate (short acting) or isosorbide mononitrate (long acting)
Calcium channel antagonists	Reduce intracellular calcium influx, therefore cardiomyocyte contraction	Nifedipine, nicardipine, amlodipine
Potassium channel blockers	Relax coronary arteries	Nicorandil
Prognostic therapies		
Cardioselective beta-blockers	Reduce sympathetic stimulation of the myocardium and reduce myocardial work	Atenolol, bisoprolol, carvedilolol
Aspirin	Reduces platelet clotting function and atherosclerotic progression	
Statins	Stabilize existing plaques by reducing blood cholesterol	Simvastatin, atorvastatin, rosuvastatin

Table 6.7 Drugs used to treat angina. NO, nitric oxide.

- **Non-ST elevation myocardial infarction** (NSTEMI): complete occlusion of a minor, or partial occlusion of a major, vessel causing infarction of a partial segment of the myocardium
- **ST elevation myocardial infarction** (STEMI): acute and complete obstruction in a main coronary artery causing infarction of a segment of the full width of the heart wall, severe pain and risk of sudden death.

Epidemiology

ACSs are rare in people under 35 years. In England, for example, there are 233600 new cases of ACS per year; about 0.6% of people aged 35–74 years and 2.3% of people aged ≥75.

Approximate annual UK incidences:
- Unstable angina: 1.15 per 1000
- NSTEMI: 3 per 1000 (also Europe)
- STEMIs: 5 per 1000.

In-hospital mortality is higher with STEMI than NSTEMI (7% versus 3–5%), although long-term (4 year) mortality is twice as high with NSTEMI, as patients are often older with significant co-morbidities.

Etiology

Etiology, and therefore primary prevention, is as for atherosclerosis and angina (see pages 172 and 226, respectively). Although there is some influence of genetic predisposition, lifestyle/environmental factors contribute to the majority of disease.

Pathogenesis

ACS tends to occur when cardiac workload increases and causes an atherosclerotic plaque to obstruct blood flow. An unstable plaque may fissure and expose the underlying lesion to blood, stimulating platelet aggregation and coagulation. The resulting thrombosis (i.e. clot) may acutely obstruct the artery, causing a sudden reduction in blood flow to the myocardium.

Myocardial infarction – and myocardial cell death – occurs if ischemia persists beyond 10 minutes. Unstable angina is ACS without infarction.

Clinical features

ACS is a clinical spectrum, though all forms usually present with angina, dyspnea and sympathetic activation (**Table 6.8**).

Symptom severity is usually: unstable angina<NSTEMI<STEMI. STEMI are the most likely to present with acute complications, including:
- Arrhythmia

Diagnosis	Exertional central chest pain relieved by GTN		Electrocardiogram		Troponin concentration	
	Yes	No	Normal	Abnormal	Normal	Increased
Angina	√		√		√	
Unstable angina		√	√		√	
NSTEMI		√		√		√
STEMI		√		√		√

Table 6.8 Diagnosis of acute coronary syndrome based on symptoms, electrocardiogram and troponin concentration. GTN, glyceryl trinitrate; NSTEMI, non-ST elevation myocardial infarction; STEMI, ST elevation myocardial infarction.

- Cardiogenic shock
- Acute heart failure.

Angina

Pain (page 90; **Figure 2.1**) in ACS is usually more severe, longer lasting, provokes more fear or occurs at a lower threshold than stable angina.

Dyspnea

The patient may feel breathless, particularly if there is pulmonary edema from left ventricular systolic impairment.

Signs

Evidence of risk factors may be present (see page 226).

Signs of sympathetic activation due to reduced cardiac output, i.e. pale and sweaty, may be seen in patients experiencing acute ischemia/infarction.

Investigations

Investigations aim to quickly distinguish angina from non-cardiac chest pain and establish and distinguish ACSs (see page 228). Patients with suspected ACS should be risk assessed in order to guide treatment.

Clinical insight

Myocardial infarction leads to sympathetic activation in response to the patient's pain, anxiety and reduced cardiac output.

ACS diagnosis requires the presence of typical ECG abnormalities (**Figure 6.2**); all patients presenting to hospital with chest pain require an ECG.

Acute MI is defined as evidence of myocardial necrosis in a clinical setting consistent with myocardial ischemia. According to the ESC, diagnosis of acute MI requires a rise and/or fall of cardiac biomarker values (ideally troponin) with one or more value above the 99th percentile of the upper reference limit and with at least one of:

- Ischemic symptoms
- New significant ST-T changes or left bundle branch block (LBBB)
- Pathological Q waves in the ECG
- A new regional wall motion abnormality seen on imaging
- Intracoronary thrombus seen on angiography.

Chest X-ray

A chest X-ray is taken to exclude pulmonary edema and aortic dissection.

Electrocardiography

Electrical evidence of arrhythmia may be present.

In unstable angina or NSTEMI, the ECG may show signs of ischemia without ST segment elevation (**Figure 6.3**). STEMI, by definition, presents with ST elevation in a pattern that reflects the myocardial territory affected (**Figure 6.1**).

Blood tests

A full blood count, urea and electrolytes test and lipid profile are needed. Cardiac markers (e.g. troponin I or T, and creatine kinase) are increased in cases of MI but normal in unstable angina.

Markers are measured at onset (if possible) and 3–6 hours after the onset of pain. The sole essential criterion for MI diagnosis is measurement of a value above the 99th percentile of the upper reference limit.

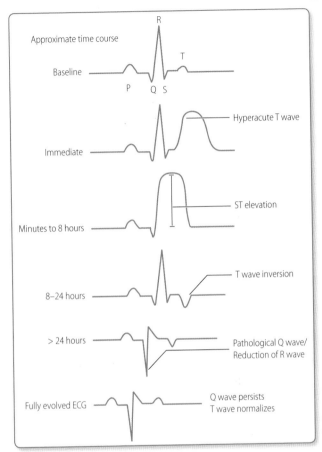

Figure 6.2 Time-dependent electrocardiograph signs of acute myocardial infarction.

Coronary angiography

Angiography shows the nature and extent of the arterial narrowing (or narrowings). Revascularization can also be performed during angiography, if indicated.

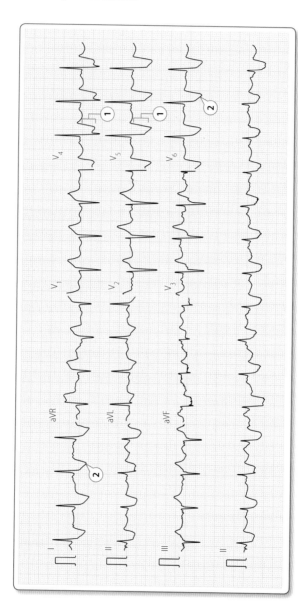

Figure 6.3 Electrocardiograph showing signs of significant myocardial ischaemia. Note the depression of the ST segments in leads I, II, aVF and V3–V6.

Management

An overview of MI management is given in **Figure 6.4**.

A central aim of managing angina or MI is to keep coronary plaques as stable as possible, using:

- Stents or grafts to reopen or bypass blocked arteries
- Anti-platelet drugs to reduce thrombosis
- Anti-cholesterol drugs to reduce atherogenesis
- Drugs to reduce myocardial oxygen demand and dilate the coronary arteries.

Lifestyle changes such as stopping smoking, reducing saturated fat intake and increasing exercise, are key in reducing the risk, and consequences, of future cardiac events (see page 306). Losing weight and increasing unsaturated fat intake will also help reduce symptom burden and improve functional capacity.

Unstable angina

Medication

- Antiplatelet and antithrombotic therapy: dual antiplatelet therapy with aspirin and another agent (i.e. clopidogrel, ticagrelor or prasugrel) are given. Patients are started on an anticoagulant such as a low-molecular weight heparin or a factor Xa inhibitor (e.g. fondaparinux), unless cardiac catheterization is planned for the same day. Unfractionated heparin is used in patients with renal impairment for closer monitoring
- Analgesics: intravenous nitrates are often required to control pain; opiates may also be required – with an appropriate antiemetic
- Secondary prevention includes treatment with a statin, an angiotensin-converting enzyme (ACE) inhibitor and a beta-blocker.

Percutaneous coronary intervention and surgery Once stabilized, patients with confirmed unstable angina undergo coronary angiography to assess and treat atherosclerotic lesions with PCI or CABG, depending on the severity and pattern of disease.

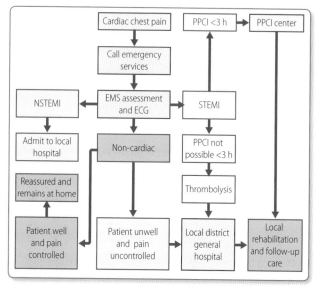

Figure 6.4 The management of myocardial infarction. ECG, electrocardiogram; EMS, emergency medical services; NSTEMI, non-ST elevation myocardial infarction; PPCI, primary percutaneous coronary intervention; STEMI, ST elevation myocardial infarction. Adapted from Boyle R. Mending hearts and brains – clinical case for change. London: Department of Health; 2006.

NSTEMI

Medication

- Antiplatelet and antithrombotic therapy: as for unstable angina (see page 239). Patients with ongoing pain and dynamic ECG changes are also given a glycoprotein IIb or IIIa inhibitor (e.g. tirofiban) to maximize blood flow through a thrombosed blood vessel and minimize further clot formation.
- Analgesics: as for unstable angina.

Percutaneous coronary intervention and surgery Patients with NSTEMI usually undergo coronary angiography within 72 h of admission to assess lesions. Once the severity and pattern of disease have been determined, the decision is made to treat the lesions medically, with stent insertion (PCI; **Figure 6.6**) or with surgery (CABG).

STEMI

It is essential that STEMI patients receive PCI as soon as possible.

> ## Clinical insight
>
> Criteria for PCI usually include chest pain <12 h in duration (from the most severe pain) and ST segment elevation of ≥1 mm in the limb leads and ≥2 mm in the chest leads, in two contiguous leads.

Medication

- Thrombolysis: can be used for patients who cannot quickly undergo PCI (door-to-balloon time <120 min). Recombinant human tissue plasminogen activator is given intravenously as soon as possible (<12 h from onset of pain). Patients need monitoring on a coronary care unit or equivalent ward. Contraindications to thrombolysis must be assessed before the drug is given.
- Antiplatelet therapy: patients are given aspirin 300 mg and another antiplatelet agent (e.g. clopidogrel 600 mg, ticagrelor 180 mg or prasugrel 60 mg according to local protocol) as soon as the diagnosis is made.

According to the 2013 ACCF/AHA and 2015 ESC guidelines, following a STEMI, all patients, assuming no contraindications, receive:

- Aspirin: required lifelong
- Additional antiplatelet agents: usually a P2Y$_{12}$ inhibitor (e.g. clopidogrel, ticagrelor or prasugrel) for ≥1 year
- Statins: to achieve target cholesterol concentrations
- ACE inhibitors and beta-blockers: to aid myocardial recovery

Percutaneous coronary intervention and surgery PCI (**Figure 2.31**) is the treatment of choice. Rarely, some patients may instead undergo CABG (**Figure 2.32**) if PCI is not suitable or if they have had an MI despite previous PCI therapy.

Prognosis

30% of patients with unstable angina will have an MI within 6 months. The mortality of NSTEMI is 2% for those that reach hospital.

Clinical insight

Door-to-balloon time is crucial for treatment of STEMI. PCI should be done within 120 min of chest pain to achieve maximum benefit.

The mortality of STEMI is 4.4% for patients who reach hospital, although 30% of patients die before reaching hospital.

STEMI patients may require subsequent coronary angiography to asses and treat further coronary lesions.

Once stable post-MI, patients require continued monitoring and treatment to assess and reduce risk of further ACS (**Table 6.6**).

6.4 Complications of myocardial infarction

MI, necrosis and scarring can lead to loss or disorder of contractility, conduction and can increase the risk of thrombosis. Many patients also have cardiac arrest after an MI. Longer term; the key complication of MI is heart failure as scarred myocardium cannot contract and cardiac output is compromised.

Arrhythmia

Arrhythmias are common but usually resolve spontaneously as tissue heals:

- Paroxysms of non-sustained ventricular tachycardia (VT) (<30 s)
- Supraventricular tachycardia (SVT)
- Accelerated idioventricular rhythm
- Ventricular ectopic beats.

Atrioventricular (AV) heart block is common in inferior territory infarcts as the posterior descending artery supplies the atrioventricular node. If it occurs due to an anterior infarct, this indicates extensive infarct territory, poor prognosis, and early pacing.

Clinical features

Patients may be asymptomatic or may experience syncope, palpitations or light-headedness. Signs include tachycardia, bradycardia and hypotension. Arrhythmia can be diagnosed from a cardiac monitoring system or ECG.

Management

Patients are best treated in a coronary care unit to diagnose and monitor arrhythmia promptly. Most resolve spontaneously within 48 h. If not, and the patient is asymptomatic, monitoring is sufficient.

The frequency of ventricular fibrillation or ventricular tachycardia can be reduced by administration of beta-blockers. If either recurs after 48 h, or if the patient is considered at high risk of future cardiac arrest (left ventricular ejection fraction <40%), they may be considered for an implantable defibrillator.

In inferior infarcts, asymptomatic, uncompromised AV block can simply be monitored, as it usually resolves spontaneously within 10 days. AV block due to an anterior infarct indicates more urgent temporary and then permanent pacing due to the poor prognosis.

Cardiac arrest

Cardiac arrest is the acute cessation of all or of effective heart contraction and is a dire emergency. Only 10% survive to be discharged.

It can occur due to an overwhelming MI, complications of an MI such as arrhythmia, or other acute or chronic heart or circulatory disease.

Clinical features

Four heart rhythms are seen:
- Ventricular tachycardia: regular rhythm, fast rate (>150 beats/min) and broad complexes
- Ventricular fibrillation: irregular rhythm, fast rate (>200 beats/min) and broad complexes
- Asystole: no rhythm, no rate and no discernible complexes
- Pulseless electrical activity: any rhythm compatible with life but without a pulse.

Only the first two are 'shockable via defibrillation'.

Management

Cardiopulmonary resuscitation (CPR) must be started immediately, as the probability of survival decreases by 10% every minute:

- A ratio of 30 chest compressions (at a depth of 6 cm and a rate of 100 per min) to 2 rescue breaths (10 per min)
- During resuscitation, assess for and treat possible reversible causes. Drugs such as adrenaline (epinephrine) and amiodarone may be required
- Early defibrillation to restart the heart is crucial.

Rupture of myocardial structures

Myocardial necrosis (particularly with severe infarcts) may result in rupture of an individual cardiac structure. This is less common when patients receive prompt and successful revascularization.

Clinical features

Rupture of the left ventricular free wall causes collapse, shock and cardiac arrest (i.e. pulseless electrical activity) and is usually rapidly fatal. An echocardiogram may show a pericardial collection of blood. Immediate surgery is indicated, but few patients survive.

Post-MI ventricular septal defect (VSD) may result from rupture of the interventricular septum or rupture of a submitral valve papillary muscle causing mitral regurgitation. This presents with features of acute heart failure and a new pansystolic murmur.

Management

Suspicion of rupture requires immediate echocardiography and referral for urgent surgical repair.

Ongoing ischemia or recurrent myocardial infarction

Post-MI patients may experience ongoing ischemia (i.e. angina), a recurrent infarction in the same territory or in a new territory. Acute stent thrombosis can occur if a clot forms inside the new stent.

Clinical features
Patients often complain of chest discomfort and are monitored with daily ECG.

Acute stent thrombosis usually presents with severe pain and ST segment elevation on ECG, in the territory of the stented artery.

Management
Urgent coronary angiography and antianginal medication (see page 162) are indicated. Angiography may indicate CABG or PCI.

Left ventricular thrombus
Scarred or akinetic myocardium can lead to clot formation on the endocardial surface, with associated risk of stroke.

Clinical features
Left ventricular thrombus is more common after an anterior territory MI and is usually identified by echocardiography.

Management
Patients require long-term anticoagulation as the lesion of scarred myocardium is permanent.

Pericarditis
Patients suffering a full-thickness MI may experience pericarditis if the infarct-related inflammation involves the pericardial membrane.

Clinical insight

A pericardial rub sounds like snow crunching underfoot.

Clinical features
Chest discomfort is the main symptom. Pericarditic pain is pleuritic in nature, and a pericardial rub may be heard on cardiac auscultation.

Management
Anti-inflammatory medications such as high-dose aspirin or colchicine are indicated and echocardiography at diagnosis and at about 7 days later is required to identify and track a pericardial effusion.

chapter 7

Arrhythmias

An arrhythmia is an abnormal heart rate or rhythm due to an abnormal generation, conduction or propagation of electrical activity. They are a heterogeneous group of conditions, and may be inconsequential, or cause syncope, cardiac arrest and death.

Coronary heart disease (CHD) is one of the principal causes of arrhythmias. Ischemia causes electrochemical instability that can initiate or compound arrhythmias. Infarction causes cardiomyocyte necrosis and scar tissue formation that can block conduction and induce or encourage arrhythmias.

In patients with CHD, arrhythmia may precipitate ischemia by increasing the metabolic demand of the myocardium. Some arrhythmias may cause thromboembolic disease . Occasionally, this can cause a blood clot to embolize to the coronary arteries causing occlusion and subsequent myocardial infarction.

Arrhythmias are categorized by heart rate, into bradycardias and tachycardias, and by the nature of the electrophysiological disturbance, for example, where the activity originates from or is localized to. Diagnosis can be difficult as many are paroxysmal in nature and there is often no correlation between symptom and pathological severity.

7.1 Clinical scenario

Lethargy and fainting

Presentation

Stan Goldman is a 72-year-old retired decorator with a long medical history of CHD, hypertension and type 2 diabetes mellitus, for which he takes diltiazem and metformin. He is seen in the outpatient clinic and gives a 4-week history of lethargy. He has 'fainted' several times, and says that 'something just isn't right'.

Diagnostic approach

Syncope (fainting) is a red flag symptom as it has serious potential cardiogenic and non-cardiogenic causes. More information is needed – most often from a collateral history – about its nature and frequency.

Further history

Mr Goldman has fainted four times in the past month, and has felt close to fainting many more times. He lacks energy and is tired all the time.

His daughter describes that he loses consciousness for a few seconds and quickly returns to normal. He has fainted whilst seated, and twice whilst standing, when he bruised and cut his limbs and head.

Examination

On examination:
- Blood pressure is 170/85 mmHg
- Radial pulse is 32 beats/min and regular.
- Jugular venous pressure is not elevated, but every few seconds a large venous pulsation is seen rising up the neck
- He has a strong, non-displaced apex beat.

The remainder of the cardiovascular and neurological examination is normal.

Diagnostic approach

His prompt recovery from loss of consciousness suggests syncope rather than seizure. Mr Goldman's marked bradycardia could indicate reduced cardiac output leading to cerebral hypoperfusion syncope.

Orthostatic hypotension is unlikely as he has been syncopal whilst sitting. His occasional large venous neck pulsation indicate atrioventricular (AV) dissociation, suggesting complete heart block.

Investigations

Blood tests confirm normal thyroid function and serum electrolytes. An urgent electrocardiogram (ECG) shows an abnormal heart rhythm (**Figure 7.1**).

Figure 7.1 Mr. Goldman's electrocardiogram, showing features of complete heart block. QRS complexes (**2**) and P waves (**1**) are both regular but occur at different rates and are dissociated from each other. The QRS complexes are broad. (**3**) points to a 'hidden' P wave occurring at the same time as a QRS complex.

> **Clinical insight**
>
> Complete heart block occurs when the ventricles receive no electrical stimulus from the atria. Endogenous ventricular pacemakers begin to pace the heart at a slower rate and more unstable rhythm (see page 34).

Diagnosis

The ECG confirms a complete heart block, warranting Mr Goldman's admission to hospital under the care of a cardiology team until a permanent pacemaker can be fitted.

In the meantime, his diltiazem is withheld (because it is a rate-limiting calcium channel blocker) and his heart rhythm is monitored in a specialist unit.

The following day, a permanent pacemaker is implanted (see page 261). Mr Goldman must not drive until he is asymptomatic for ≥4 weeks.

Mr Goldman has CHD which is a risk factor for heart block. His calcium channel blocker (diltiazem) has not caused the CHB, but will only compound the situation and must be withheld.

7.2 Mechanisms of arrhythmia

Arrhythmias are aberrations of normal cardiac electrophysiology (see page 28).

Conduction block

Any disease that reduces conduction velocity or blocks it altogether causes bundle branch block, bradycardia or heart block (see page 256). Causes include:

- Ischemia or infarction – the most common cause
- Infiltrative disease, e.g. amyloid disease
- Surgery
- Drugs.

The clinical effect depends on the nature and location of the block, which is diagnosed by ECG rhythm and QRS morphology.

Ectopic beats

An ectopic beat is an 'extra' heartbeat (or 'extrasystole') initiated outside of the region where impulse formation is ordinarily generated, i.e. the the sino-atrial (SA) node. They occur when cardiomyocyte auto-maticity increases causing premature discharge.

Occasional ectopics are normal but their frequency can increase due to:

> ## Clinical insight
>
> Drugs that reduce AVN conduction velocity (e.g. Ca^{2+} channel blockers, β-blockers and digoxin) should be avoided in patients with significant conduction deficit as they may compound it.

- Ischemia causing electrolyte derangement and sympathetic activation (**Figure 7.2**)
- Electrolyte derangement
- Sympathetic activation
- Myocardial stretch
- Drugs that disrupt the resting membrane potential and/or alter ion channel function.

The more distal the site, the less coordinated its propagation through the conduction pathway. Atrial ectopics, therefore, cause abnormal P wave morphology on the ECG, whereas ventricular ectopics result in a broad QRS complex with abnormal morphology.

Re-entry

A conduction re-entry circuit is an alternative, abnormal route of cardiac conduction that loops back on itself. This can lead to

Figure 7.2 Re-entry. An impulse arrives at an area of scar tissue ①. It is blocked on one side ② but can pass on the other. Part of the signal then conducts retrogradely around the scar ③. If this conduction is slow enough (dashed line), by the time it reaches ④ the myocardium can be depolarized again and the re-entry circuit continues.

a cyclic conduction of varying duration that disrupts the heart rate and rhythm. Re-entry circuits require:

- A circuit of conducting tissue
- An area of the circuit where conduction is unidirectional
- Timing: conduction is slow enough to allow time for local cardiomyocyte repolarization, but is faster than the normal conduction pathway.

A circuit is often instigated by scar tissue formation, most commonly the result of infarction (**Figure 7.2**). The property of electrophysiological timing means any factor that influences conduction velocity and/or repolarization time will effect whether the re-entry occurs or not. Re-entry is a cause of supraventricular tachycardia (SVT) and ventricular tachycardia (VT).

Triggered activity and after-depolarizations

Premature depolarizations can occur during phase 3 or 4 of repolarization to cause an irregular heartbeat. An arrhythmia, e.g. torsade de pointes, can arise if these depolarizations recur regularly.

In the acute phases of ischemia and myocardial infarction, triggered activity is increased (see **Figure 7.2**) which adds to the pro-arrhythmic milieu.

Early after-depolarizations (EADs) occur in phase 3 and delayed after-depolarizations (DADs) in phase 4. EADs are more common if phase 3 repolarization is prolonged, for example in long QT syndrome or with certain drugs. DADs are more common with increased cytoplasmic Ca^{2+} concentrations, as occurs in sympathetic activation.

CHD arrhythmogenesis

Myocardial ischemia and infarction are common causes of arrhythmias by disrupting cardiac electrophysiology and/or conduction pathways (**Table 7.1** and **Figures 7.2** and **7.3**).

Acute myocardial ischemia is the most common cause of ventricular tachycardia or fibrillation leading to sudden cardiac death.

Ischemia

Ischemia causes evolving changes in electrochemistry inside and outside of cells. It is also associated with sympathetic activation, which is arrhythmogenic.

Electrochemistry

Extracellular changes include: raised K^+ and adenosine concentrations, increased lactate and CO_2 production (and resulting acidosis), and catecholamine release. Intracellular changes include: acidosis, elevated cyclic adenosine monophosphate (cAMP), Ca^{2+}, Mg^{2+}, and Na^+.

These changes alter ionic membrane transport, causing disruption of cardiomyocyte resting membrane and action potential including:

- Decreased excitability
- Slowed conduction
- Shorter action potential duration
- Depolarization of the resting membrane potential
- Abnormal automaticity.

Sympathetic activation

Triggered by ischemia, pain and anxiety, autonomic sympathetic activation causes increases in:

- Junctional and Purkinje fiber automaticity
- Re-entry circuits during acute myocardial ischemia
- After-depolarizations during phase 2, 3, or 4
- Risk of ventricular fibrillation.

It is associated with ECG changes in P wave morphology, and shorter QT and PR intervals.

Infarction

Myocardial infarction (MI) leads to cardiomyocyte necrosis, scar tissue formation (fibrosis) and sympathetic activation.

Fibrosis causes electrical conduction to slow or change route, increasing the risk of re-entry circuits and unsynchronized ventricular contraction.

Arrhythmias caused by myocardial infarction:

Arrhythmia	Prevalence	Timing/mechanism	Significance
Ventricular tachycardia	Non-sustained VT ~10% Sustained VT ~1% Polymorphic VT ~1%	2–10 min – altered cellular electrophysiology and re-entry 10–30 min – catecholamine driven and increased automaticity ≤72 hrs (peak 12–24 h) – increased automaticity, triggered activity, re-entry mechanisms >72 h – primarily re-entrant mechanisms	Immediately post-infarct, non-sustained VT is associated with a 2× risk of cardiac arrest. In the presence of LVSD, this increases to 5× Sustained VT is uncommon in the peri-infarct period, it usually indicates previous MI/scarring. Polymorphic VT usually reflects ongoing or recurrent ischemia. Prognosis similar to sustained VT. Both are associated with increased in-hospital mortality
Ventricular fibrillation	~3%	60% of episodes occur ≤4 h and 80% ≤12 h	Rapidly fatal without prompt defibrillation
Accelerated idioventricular rhythm	~40%	Due to an ectopic ventricular focus firing at <120 bpm but faster than the sinus node rate Common in first 24 h post successful re-perfusion	Usually benign. Does not influence long term prognosis
Sinus bradycardia	~30%	Commonly within 1 h	More common in inferior wall infarcts, secondary to hypervagotonia
Sinus tachycardia	~30%	Peri-infarct period, within 72 h	Aggravates myocardial ischaemia. Can indicate underlying ventricular dysfunction

Table 7.1 *Continued*

Arrhythmia	Prevalence	Timing / mechanism	Significance
Supraventricular tachycardias	AF ~ 10% AFL ~ 5%	Mostly within 72 h. AF occurring within 24 h often associated with inferior infarction. AF occurring > 24 h often associated with anterior wall infarction and LVSD	AF is associated with increased in-hospital and long-term mortality, re-infarction, ventricular arrhythmias, cardiac arrest, shock, strokes and may reflect extensive CAD and insufficient reperfusion
AV conduction block	1st degree ~15% 2nd degree ~10% Complete ~ 5%	Most occur in peri-infarct period. AV block is commoner in inferior wall infarcts reflecting hypervagotonia or damage to the AV node	AV block indicates a poorer prognosis in the context of anterior wall infarcts

Table 7.1 Prevalence, mechanism and timing of arrhythmias occurring after myocardial infarction. VT, ventricular tachycardia; LVSD, left ventricular systolic dysfunction; MI, myocardial infarction; AF, atrial fibrillation; AFL, atrial flutter; CAD, coronary artery disease; AV, atrioventricular. Adapted from Data from Ghuran AV, Camm J. Br Med Bull 2001.

Figure 7.3 The pathophysiological mechanisms of arrhythmia in coronary heart disease. Catecholamines and arrhythmia itself can both exacerbate ischaemia by increasing the metabolic demands of the myocardium.

7.3 Bradyarrhythmias

Bradycardia is a ventricular rate <60 bpm whereas a bradyarrhythmia is an inappropriately slow ventricular rhythm. They reflect a reduction in either electrical activity or conduction.

Myocardial ischemia can produce a variety of conduction disturbances affecting any component or level of the conduction pathway. More chronically, CHD can cause fibrosis and dysfunction of the conduction tissues leading to a number of bradyarrhythmias.

Etiology

Table 7.2 lists some common non-cardiac causes of bradycardia. Specific cardiac bradyrrhythmic syndromes include sinus node disease, heart block, atrial fibrillation (AF) and chronotropic incompetence. CHD is a major cause and should be considered in all patients presenting with bradyarrhythmia.

Sinus node disease

Sinus node dysfunction can cause:

- Sinus pauses – temporary absence or delay of SA node impulse generation
- Sinus tachycardia
- Sinus bradycardia
- Atrial tachycardia
- Chronotropic incompetence (see page 258)
- AF.

Tachy–brady syndrome is episodes of bradycardia and atrial tachycardia in the same patient, and suggests sinus node disease.

Physiological	Sleep
	Athletic training (increased vagal tone)
Drug effects	Beta-blockers
	Calcium channel blockers (dihydropyridine class)
	Amiodarone
Metabolic	Hypothyroidism
	Hypothermia
Electrolyte disturbance	Deranged potassium
	Deranged calcium
	Deranged magnesium
	Deranged sodium
Others	Increased intracranial pressure
	Obstructive sleep apnea

Table 7.2 Common non-cardiac causes of bradycardia and bradyarrhythmia

Heart block

Heart block is impaired conduction between the atria and the ventricles. It is categorized by severity into 1st, 2nd and 3rd degree – or complete – heart block (**Table 7.3** and **Figure 7.4**).

All cases of complete heart block require urgent specialist referral due to the increased risk of asystole. The slower the ventricular escape rate and the broader the QRS complexes, the more unstable the rhythm.

Atrial fibrillation

AF (see page 275) can be associated with a bradycardic ventricular response, especially in the context of rate limiting drug therapy. The rhythm is irregular, but the rate depends on the ventricular response.

Chronotropic incompetence

This occurs when a patient's heart rate fails to rise appropriately with exercise or physiological stress. It is often diagnosed with exercise ECG testing.

Degree	ECG features	Treatment
1st	Prolonged PR interval	Conservative
2nd	Prolonging PR interval culminating in a dropped ventricular beat (QRS complex)	Conservative
	Regularly more than one P wave to each QRS complex in a 2:1, 3:1 or 4:1 ratio; higher levels of block and variable block are also possible	Permanent pacemaker if symptomatic*
3rd (complete)	Complete atrioventricular dissociation: regular P waves, regular QRS complexes and no association between the two	Permanent pacemaker*

Table 7.3 Types of heart block, their features on electrocardiography and treatment.* If reversible causes are excluded.

Figure 7.4 Electrocardiographic features of heart block. (a) 1st-degree heart block: a prolonged PR interval. (b) A 2nd-degree heart block (Mobitz type 1, Wenckebach block): progressive prolongation of the PR interval culminates in a dropped QRS complex. (c) A 2nd-degree heart block (Mobitz type 2, with 2:1 block): there is an absence of the QRS complex after alternate P waves. (d) A 3rd-degree (complete) heart block: dissociated atrial and ventricular activity.

Chronotropic incompetence causes symptoms on exertion and may be the first sign of another bradyarrhythmia. If it is sufficiently symptomatic, a permanent pacemaker may be indicated.

Pathophysiology

Bradycardia is caused by conditions that reduce automaticity or block conduction tissues via infiltrative or fibrotic disease including:

- CHD
- Age-related fibrosis
- Myocardial infiltration (sarcoidosis and amyloidosis)
- Rheumatoid conditions (systemic lupus erythematosus and rheumatoid arthritis)
- Congenital heart disease
- Electrolyte disturbance (e.g. hyperkalemia)
- Hypothyroidism
- Excessive vagal tone
- Heart surgery.

Clinical features

Bradycardia causes palpitations, light-headedness and dizziness (non-vertiginous). Systolic blood pressure (pulse pressure) is often increased in the early stages. Significant symptoms are unusual unless the heart rate is <45 beats/min. Severe bradycardia results in collapse and syncope.

Hypotension, cerebral hypoperfusion (resulting in confusion) and shock indicate cardiovascular decompensation, a late and dangerous sign.

Diagnostic approach

Diagnosis relies on ECG to 'catch' the arrhythmia when it occurs. Less frequent paroxysmal bradycardias can therefore be difficult to diagnose.

Investigations

Blood tests are done to exclude a biochemical cause (**Table 7.2**).

A 12-lead ECG may detect more frequent bradyarrhythmias, otherwise, ambulatory ECG may be needed.

Management

Asymptomatic bradycardia is usually treated conservatively, unless there is a compelling reason to insert a permanent pacemaker such as complete heart block.

For symptomatic bradyarrhythmia, reversible secondary causes such as drugs should first be excluded. Otherwise, a pacemaker is usually indicated.

Pacemakers

Definitive treatment for symptomatic bradycardia is permanent pacemaker implantation (**Figure 7.5**). Implantation is not

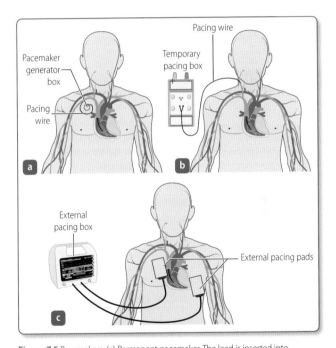

Figure 7.5 Pacemakers. (a) Permanent pacemaker. The lead is inserted into the right ventricle via a central vein and the generator box is inserted into a subcutaneous pocket. (b) Temporary transvenous pacing. A wire is inserted into the right ventricle under X-ray imaging through the jugular, subclavian or femoral vein. The wire is then connected to a generator box outside the body. (c) Transcutaneous pacing. Electrical activity is delivered through pads on the anterior chest wall.

Complication	Context
Pneumothorax	Occurs if a lung pleura is damaged during insertion
Bleeding	Post-procedural pocket haematoma – usually treated with a compression dressing in the first instance
Perforation	Can result in cardiac tamponade (i.e. compression of the heart by fluid build-up within the pericardial space), which requires emergency drainage
Infection	Treatment involves long courses of intravenous antibiotics and extraction of the pacemaker if this is unsuccessful (a risky procedure)
Lead displacement	Causes device to malfunction, requires lead repositioning

Table 7.4 Complications of permanent pacemaker insertion.

Clinical insight

Rate-limiting drugs (e.g. calcium-channel blockers; see page 156) should usually be withheld during symptomatic bradyarrhythmia.

without risk (**Table 7.4**) and so requires that:

- Reversible causes have been excluded
- Symptoms are proven to be secondary to bradycardia
- Any infection is eradicated before insertion.

Emergency and interim treatment

Severe bradycardia causing acute cardiac instability is an indication for temporary pacing or infusion with an intravenous (IV) chronotropic drug until a permanent pacemaker system can be implanted (**Figure 7.4**).

Transvenous pacing involves inserting a pacing wire into the right ventricular apex through a central vein and pacing the heart from an external power box.

An IV infusion of a positive chronotrope such as isoprenaline or atropine can be used (in specialist units with cardiac monitoring) to stabilize the patient once ischemia is excluded.

Cardiac pauses

A cardiac pause is a transient cessation in cardiac electrical activity due to impulse conduction failure at the SA node, in

Type	Cause	Features
Sinus arrest	Temporary cessation of SA node impulse formation	No evidence of atrial activity (i.e. absent P waves) Duration is independent of the normal P–P interval
SA block	Transient failure of conduction across the atrial myocardium	Length of two or more times the normal P–P interval
AV block	Temporary block of AV node conduction.	Atrial depolarization (P waves) may not be followed by ventricular depolarization. A pause in cardiac output occurs before either AV conduction is restored or a ventricular escape rhythm occurs

Table 7.5 Causes and features of cardiac pauses

3.4s pause

Figure 7.6
Electrocardiogram showing a cardiac pause of 3.4 s. The rest of the electrocardiogram shows normal sinus rhythm.

the atrial myocardium or at the AV node (**Table 7.5**, **Figure 7.6**). The clinical features, diagnostic approach and management are similar to those for other paroxysmal bradyarrhythmias.

Clinical features
Pauses result in a pause in cardiac output that is usually asymptomatic but may cause palpitations, transient light-headedness and, occasionally, syncope.

Investigations
Pauses are best identified via Holter ECG monitoring (see page 133).

Clinical insight

Holter ECG monitoring usually lasts 24–72 hours and involves a 'patient symptom diary'. This allows clinicians to interpret the ECG in line with concurrent symptoms. Symptoms that occur during normal sinus rhythm do not respond to pacemaker insertion.

Waking pauses lasting over 3 seconds are considered significant and require further investigation, especially when accompanied by symptoms.

7.4 Tachyarrhythmias

Tachycardia is a ventricular rate >100 bpm whereas a tachyarrhythmia is an abnormally fast ventricular rhythm.

Tachyarrhythmias are categorized by the duration of the QRS complex (**Table 7.6**).

Narrow complex tachycardias reflect organized, efficient electrical conduction originating from above the AV node. They are often stable and benign. Broad complex tachycardias may reflect an origin below the AV node (ventricular tachycardias) or a supraventricular origin with aberrant conduction, e.g. bundle branch block. Ventricular tachycardias are less stable and can be associated with cardiac arrest.

CHD is a major cause of supraventricular and ventricular arrhythmias both in the acute and chronic phases. Investigations for CHD should be considered in all patients presenting with tachyarrhythmias.

Supraventricular/narrow complex tachyarrhythmias

Supraventricular/narrow complex tachyarrhythmias are arrhythmias with tachycardia and a QRS duration <120 ms.

Type	QRS duration	Origin	Electrical activity
Narrow complex (or supraventricular) tachyarrythmias	≤120 ms	Above the AV node	Organised, efficient
Broad complex tachyarrythmias	>120 ms	Below the AV node*	Unstable/ disorganised, delayed depolarization

Table 7.6 Narrow and broad complex tachyarrythmias. * unless supraventricular with aberrant conduction, e.g. bundle branch block.

They can be asymptomatic or symptomatic. In an otherwise healthy heart, they are usually a relatively benign problem. AF is the most common type (see page 275).

Modern catheter-based treatments that ablate the abnormal conduction tissue offer a high chance of a cure.

Epidemiology

Supraventricular tachycardias (SVTs) affect about 0.2% of the population.

Etiology

SVTs are categorized by the nature and location of the electrophysiological abnormality.

> **Guiding principle**
>
> Accessory pathways are embryological artifacts leaving conductible tissue through the fibrous cartilage that separates the atria and ventricles.

Atrioventricular nodal re-entry tachycardia

50% of SVTs are caused by a small re-entry circuit involving the AV node and surrounding atrial tissue. ECG characteristics of atrioventricular nodal re-entry tachycardia are shown in **Figure 7.7**.

Although the abnormality is present at birth (i.e. it is congenital), symptoms usually do not occur until young adulthood. Heart rates are usually 140–220 bpm.

Atrioventricular reciprocating tachycardia

Approximately 30% of SVTs are caused by an accessory pathway (AP), an abnormal electrical connection between atria and ventricle which may conduct in either direction (A-V or V-A). APs cause arrhythmia if the abnormal circuit usurps the normal conduction sequence. The resulting arrhythmia may

Figure 7.7 Electrocardiographic features of atrioventricular node re-entry tachycardia. Note the tachycardia and narrow QRS complexes. The atria and ventricles depolarise almost synchronously so that P waves are hidden inside the QRS complexes.

be narrow or broad complex depending on the direction of conduction:

- Narrow complex tachycardia occurs when the circuit conducts down the AV node and septum in an antegrade (i.e. forward, normal or orthodromic) direction and the AP conducts from ventricle to atrium (**Figure 7.8**)
- Broad complex tachycardia results when the AP conducts from atrium to ventricle and there is retrograde (i.e. reverse or antidromic) conduction along the septum and through the AV node.

APs are present from birth and usually manifest from childhood or adolescence.

Wolff–Parkinson–White (WPW) syndrome This is when there is evidence of ventricular pre-excitation caused by an AP conducting in the A-V direction. Premature ventricular excitation causes a shortened PR interval and a slurring of the R wave upstroke, i.e. a 'delta wave' (**Figure 7.9**). WPW syndrome predisposes to AVRT (and AF) but can be asymptomatic in up to 50%.

> ## Clinical insight
>
> In atrioventricular reciprocating tachycardias, the breadth of QRS is determined by the direction of the circuit. Orthodromic conduction is antegrade down the septum and ventricles. Antidromic is more abnormal because conduction goes the 'wrong' way around the ventricles and the wrong way up the septum – this is inefficient and broadens the QRS.

Atrial flutter

Atrial flutter (AFL) is a macro re-entry arrhythmia within the atria. Typical AFL circuits involve the cavotricuspid isthmus, atrial septum and the crista terminalis resulting in an atrial rate

Figure 7.8 Electrocardiographic features of orthodromic atrioventricular reciprocating tachycardia. The atria are depolarised by the ventricles through an accessory pathway resulting in a retrograde P wave (arrow) after a narrow QRS complex.

Figure 7.9
Electrocardiographic features of Wolff-Parkinson-White syndrome. The short PR interval and slurring of the QRS upstroke (delta wave) indicate early ventricular depolarization through the accessory pathway during sinus rhythm.

of around 300 bpm. Atypical AFL circuits occur elsewhere in the atria, and usually associated with previous surgery or scarring.

Flutter is usually episodic (but can be chronic) and presents with tachycardia of around 150 bpm (when there is 2:1 block) and a classical saw-tooth appearance on ECG as seen in **Figure 7.10**.

Atrial tachycardia

This SVT arises from increased automaticity, a macro or micro re-entry circuit, or both, in the atria. It causes a narrow complex tachycardia with an abnormal P wave shape.

Guiding principle

Despite atrial contractions of around 250–300 bpm in AFL, the AV node limits conduction to the ventricles, resulting in a ventricular rate of 75, 100 or 150 bpm, i.e. a value divisible into 300.

Atrial fibrillation

AF consists of fast, disorganized atrial impulses that – unlike other SVTs – causes an irregularly irregular rhythm (see page 275). AF occurs with either a normal, slow or fast ventricular response rate.

Figure 7.10
Electrocardiogram showing atrial flutter. Note the sawtooth baseline (blue) and narrow complex tachycardia (100 bpm). There are three flutter waves to each QRS but the third is hidden within the QRS complex.

Clinical features

SVTs may be asymptomatic or cause:
- Fast, regular or 'fluttering' palpitations
- Shortness of breath
- Fatigue.

Ischaemic chest pain and low blood pressure indicate myocardial compromise and require urgent (synchronised) direct current cardioversion (DCCV) to correct the arrhythmia.

Tachycardiomyopathy is heart failure due to persistent SVT. It develops over weeks or months. SVTs are much more often a complication of, and not the cause of, heart failure.

Investigations

Diagnosis relies on defining the SVT on ECG and correlating it with patient symptoms. Ambulatory ECG monitoring may be required if episodes are infrequent.

Once diagnosed, investigations are used to identify the cause (**Table 7.7**).

Investigation	Rationale
Echocardiography	Excludes structural heart disease and assess cardiac function
Thyroid function tests	Hyperthyroidism
Urea and electrolytes	Electrolyte derangement
Invasive electrophysiological studies	Characterize underlying pathophysiology
Investigations for CHD, e.g. coronary angiography (page 228)	If ischemia is suspected as a precipitant

Table 7.7 Investigations in supraventricular tachycardia.

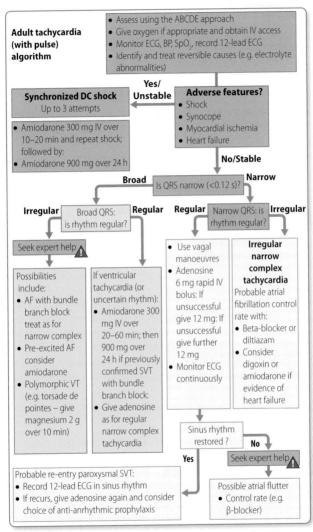

Figure 7.11 Advanced support guidelines for the management of tachycardia. AF, atrial fibrillation; BP, blood pressure; DC, direct current; ECG, electrocardiogram; IV, intravenous; SpO₂, oxygen saturation; SVT, supraventricular tachycardia; VT, ventricular tachycardia. Reproduced with the kind permission of the Resuscitation Council (UK).

Management

SVTs causing cardiovascular instability indicate urgent synchronized DCCV (**Figure 7.11**).

Ultimately, the optimal management is determined by the underlying cause. Drug therapy may reduce the chance of recurrence, whereas catheter ablation offers the possibility of a cure.

Vagal manoeuvers

Vagal stimulation may terminate a SVT quickly and simply. These include:

- The Valsalva manoeuvre – ask the patient to cough, bear down or blow hard into a 10 mL syringe
- Carotid sinus massage – after carotid bruit is excluded.

> **Clinical insight**
>
> Atrial flutter, like AF, often requires thromboprophylaxis due to increased stroke risk due to increased blood stasis (see page 150).

Medication

Drugs that block AV node conduction (e.g. β-blockers and Ca^{2+} channel blockers) are effective in treating AV node re-entry and AV reciprocating tachycardias. They are contraindicated if ventricular pre-excitation is evident (e.g. in Wolff–Parkinson–White syndrome), because they increase the accessory pathway conduction causing pre-excitation. Instead, class 1 (flecanide, propafenone or disopyramide) or class 3 drugs (amiodarone) are favored, as they reduce accessory pathway conduction.

Atrial flutter and atrial tachycardia respond poorly to drug therapy.

> **Clinical insight**
>
> Always consider atrial flutter if the ventricular rate is 150. The atrial rate in flutter is always about 300, which is too fast for 1:1 AV node conduction. Ventricular rate usually occurs with 2:1 (150 beats/min), 3:1 (100 beats/min) or 4:1 (75 beats/min) AV block.

Catheter ablation

Either cryotherapy or radiofrequency ablation is the destruction of the abnormal circuit or electrical focus causing the tachycardia. It is delivered through intracardiac catheters and has a high success rate (>95%).

Prognosis

Although SVT may be worrying and difficult to treat, in an otherwise healthy heart, the prognosis is usually excellent.

Ventricular tachycardia

Ventricular tachycardia (VT) is a broad complex tachycardia originating in the ventricular myocardium. It is defined as ≥3 successive ventricular beats occurring at >100 bpm.

VT is potentially life threatening, due to the risk of ventricular fibrillation, cardiac arrest, and sudden cardiac death.

> ## Clinical insight
>
> Not all supraventricular tachycardias (SVT) present with a narrow complex; some can present with broad QRS complexes:
>
> - SVT with abnormal conduction, e.g. atrial flutter with bundle branch block, can present with a regular broad complex tachycardia
> - AF with a fast ventricular response and abnormal conduction (i.e. left or right bundle branch block) presents with an irregular broad complex tachycardia.

Types

VT may be:
- Pulse-palpable or pulseless
- Non-sustained (<30 s) or sustained (>30 s)
- Monomorphic (with a consistent QRS appearance; **Figure 7.12**) or polymorphic (with a frequently changing QRS appearance; **Figure 7.13**)

Etiology

Monomorphic ventricular tachycardias are usually caused by

Figure 7.12 Electrocardiographic features of a regular broad complex ventricular tachycardia.

Figure 7.13 Electrocardiogram features of torsade de pointes, a polymorphic broad complex tachycardia. The complexes appear to twist around the baseline.

an abnormal re-entry circuit, often due to myocardial scarring secondary to CHD. Other causes include infiltration or cardiomyopathy.

Torsades de pointes is a polymorphic ventricular tachycardia that occurs secondary to prolonged QT interval. It is therefore associated with the long QT syndromes, hypokalemia and hypomagnesemia, as well as the use of amiodarone, erythromycin and methadone.

Clinical features

VT is usually symptomatic. Symptoms include:

- Palpitations
- Presyncope – lightheadedness, blurred vision, weakness.
- Syncope, i.e. loss of consciousness. This is a poor prognostic indicator
- Symptoms of heart failure in sustained ventricular tachycardia.

Patients are often agitated, anxious and fatigued.

History should also elicit symptoms of associated conditions, such as CHD and heart failure. Family history of arrhythmia or sudden cardiac death is also relevant.

If palpable, the pulse is usually rapid and weak. Pulseless ventricular tachycardia presents with cardiac arrest. Signs of potential causes or complications should also be sought.

Investigations

VT is diagnosed by 12 lead ECG and must be distinguished from broad-complex SVTs (**Table 7.8**). About 85% of regular broad complex tachycardias are caused by VT. In patients with structural heart disease (including heart failure or CHD), around 95% of broad complex tachycardias are caused by VT. Therefore, in cases of doubt, the arrhythmia is treated as VT until proven otherwise.

Underlying cause

The underlying cause may be evident on ECG or cardiac magnetic resonance imaging (cMRI), which can show functional impairment or structural abnormalities, and coronary

	Ventricular tachycardia	SVT with aberrant conduction
QRS complex	Very broad QRS: >160 ms	<160 ms
Axis	Extreme: −90° to −180°	Normal QRS axis (−30 – +90°)
Concordance	All chest lead complexes are positive or all are negative	Not present
Fusion beats	Produced when a sinus beat fuses with a ventricular beat	Not present
Capture beats	Produced when a sinus beat 'captures' the ventricles to produce occasional 'normal'-looking beats	Not present
Bizarre QRS shapes	Present	Not present
AV dissociation	AV dissociation: regular P and QRS complexes but at different rates	Not present

Table 7.8 Typical ECG features of VT and SVT with aberrant conduction. The latter occurs when there is a SVT with abnormal and prolonged conduction between the atria and ventricles, e.g. bundle branch block.

angiography may be used to diagnose CHD.

Electrophysiology

The mechanism of the arrhythmia can be identified through an invasive electrophysiological study. Multiple catheters are positioned within the heart and coronary sinus to detect the electrical activation sequence. This helps determine the underlying electrical abnormality and guides ablation therapy.

Clinical insight

Accelerated idioventricular rhythms are ventricular in origin with a rate between 60–100 bpm. They are commonly associated with successful reperfusion following treatment for myocardial infarction. In this context, they usually resolve spontaneously.

Quantifying risk

Risk is determined by the presence or absence of structural heart disease, including heart failure and CHD.

Management

Emergency synchronized DCCV is required for any patient whose condition is acutely compromised, for example, hypotension or ischemia.

Once sinus rhythm is restored, the underlying cause is sought and treated where possible. This commonly requires alleviating ischemia or optimising treatment of heart failure.

Torsades de pointes requires urgent DCCV to restore sinus rhythm. Correction of magnesium or potassium deficiency, or both, in addition to cessation of any QT-prolonging drugs reduces recurrence.

Medication

Drugs (e.g. amiodarone or β-blockers) may be used to reduce the frequency of VT in patients with a structurally abnormal heart. β-blockers and aldosterone antagonists may improve prognosis in the context of heart failure.

In patients with a structurally normal heart, drug therapy is often the only management necessary.

Surgery

If electrophysiological investigations identify an appropriate target, catheter ablation may be possible for monomorphic VT. Success rates are about 60–75%, and higher in the absence of structural abnormality.

Cardioverter defibrillators

Implantable cardioverter defibrillators (ICDs), after careful consideration, are used for primary prevention in patients with a high-risk condition (e.g. severe heart failure) and secondary prevention in patients with VT or VF causing syncope or cardiac arrest.

ICDs do not reduce the frequency of ventricular arrhythmia, but attempt to restore sinus rhythm when it occurs.

Prognosis

The key prognostic factor is the presence of structural heart disease, including CHD and heart failure. VT in a structurally normal heart has a much better prognosis. In appropriate patients, ICD insertion has been shown to reduce mortality.

Figure 7.14
Electrocardiographic features of ventricular fibrillation. The rhythm, polarity and magnitude are completely irregular.

Ventricular fibrillation

In VF, the ventricular myocardium is devoid of any coordinated electrical or mechanical activity. Cardiac output ceases and cardiac arrest occurs (**Figure 7.14**). Immediate DCCV is indicated in all cases otherwise asystole and death quickly ensue. Survival is highly dependent on speed and quality of advanced life support treatment and defibrillation. Survival probability declines 2–10% per minute of delay of DCCV.

VF survivors and those deemed to be at high risk of VF are treated with ICD implantation.

7.5 Atrial fibrillation

AF is an irregular, often rapid rhythm where the atria fail to contract efficiently, regularly or in coordination with the ventricles. It is the commonest cardiac arrhythmia. Depending on the ventricular response rate, it can present with bradycardia, tachycardia, or a normal rate.

AF is a major risk factor for thromboembolic disease, especially stroke, as it increases blood clotting due to stasis. AF often occurs in patients with CHD and may complicate the acute or chronic phases of myocardial infarction.

Types

AF is classed according to duration:
- Paroxysmal (<7 days)
- Persistent (>7 days)
- Permanent (>7 days and resistant to therapy).

Epidemiology

AF prevalence increases with age. It affects 1% of the general population and up to 10% of those over 80. Its true prevalence is likely higher than this as it is often asymptomatic and undiagnosed.

Etiology

AF can be:

- Lone, with no identifiable cause (10–15%)
- Valvular, often associated with prosthetic valves or rheumatic valve disease
- Secondary to other cardiac or non-cardiac disease that increases atrial stress (**Table 7.9**).

Excess alcohol consumption and drug misuse also predispose to AF. It is common in the acutely unwell or perioperative patients.

Pathophysiology

Fibrillation is a pattern of rapid, unsynchronized electrical activity, with no coordination of atrial electrical or mechanical

Common risk factors	Common investigative findings
CHD (including previous MI)	LVH (ECG or echo)
Valvular heart disease	Dilated left atrium (echo)
Heart failure	Valve (particularly mitral) dysfunction (echo)
Advanced age	Systolic or diastolic dysfunction (echo)
Obesity	Raised inflammatory markers (serum CRP/ESR)
Hypertension	Elevated white cell count
Diabetes mellitus	
Previous cardiac surgery	
Smoking	
Alcohol excess	
Hyperthyroidism	
Family history	

Table 7.9 Common risk factors for and investigation findings in atrial fibrillation. CHD, coronary heart disease; MI, myocardial infarction; LVH, left ventricular hypertrophy; MI, myocardial infarction; and VHD, valvular heart disease.

activity. Conduction to the ventricles is irregular and haphazard, so the ventricular response rate is determined by the conductivity of the AV node and the His and Purkinje tissues.

The mechanisms of AF initiation and propagation are complex and not fully understood, but involve structural and electrophysiological alterations of the atrial tissue caused by a spectrum of pathological mechanisms including ischemia, inflammation, increased metabolic demand and neurohormonal activation. AF is often the final common result of a variety of disease processes.

Clinical insight

Atrial stress induces chronic myocardial, electrical and biochemical changes that initiate and propagate AF. In many patients with paroxysmal AF, the initiating electrical stimuli emanate from the pulmonary veins. This is the rationale behind pulmonary vein ablation (isolation) therapy in paroxysmal AF (see page 281).

Clinical features

The clinical features of AF are often determined by the ventricular response rate. However, even AF with normal ventricular rate may be symptomatic with palpitations, lethargy, chest pain and dyspnoea. In otherwise asymptomatic cases, the first presentation can be with a cerebrovascular accident.

History should also include:
- Predisposing factors (e.g. family history, hypertension and lung disease)
- Stroke and bleeding risk
- Complications (e.g. heart failure and thromboembolic disease).

Signs include:
- An irregularly irregular pulse
- Those of predisposing factors (see **Table 7.9**)
- Complications – e.g. signs of heart failure or thromboembolic disease.

Clinical insight

Atrial fibrillation is always 'fast': it is the ventricular response rate that can be slow, normal or fast.

Clinical insight

Atrial fibrillation predisposes blood clots, often in the left atrial appendage. These are best seen via transoesophageal echocardiography

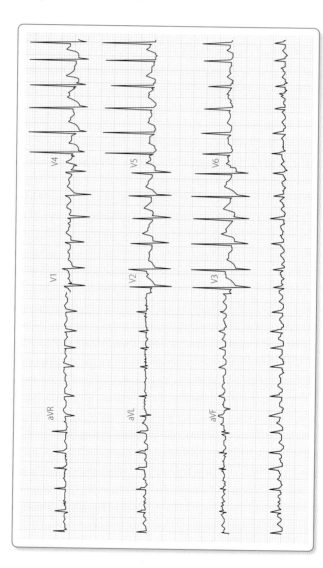

Figure 7.15 Electrocardiographic features of atrial fibrillation. The QRS complexes are narrow and occur irregularly irregularly. P waves are absent.

Investigations

Permanent AF is easily and quickly diagnosed by palpating an irregularly irregular pulse rhythm and performing an ECG (**Figure 7.15**). Paroxysmal AF usually requires Holter monitoring to record an episode.

Multiple investigations are necessary to exclude causes and guide treatment (**Table 7.10**). Transoesophageal echocardiography can also be done to identify or exclude left atrial clot if DCCV is being considered in AF beyond 48 h and before 6 weeks of anticoagulation is complete.

Management

The key aims are to reduce the risk of thromboembolic disease, control the ventricular rate and alleviate symptoms. The strategy depends on whether AF is acute, paroxysmal or permanent.

Anticoagulation AF increases the risk of stroke five-fold. This risk is decreased by around two thirds by oral anticoagulant therapy. Annual risk should be calculated using, for example, the CHA_2DS_2-VASc score (**Table 7.11**). The patient's risk of bleeding, calculated with, for example, the HAS-BLED score, must be balanced against the benefits of anticoagulation.

Rate control The initial target is maintenance of a resting heart rate ≤110 beats/min, using a beta-blocker, calcium channel-

Test	Rationale
Thyroid function tests	To exclude hyperthyroidism
Coagulation screen	Required for patients considered for anticoagulation
Urea and electrolytes	To exclude electrolyte derangement
Liver function tests	To exclude derangement and assess clotting function
Echocardiography	To exclude structural heart disease

Table 7.10 Investigations indicated by atrial fibrillation.

Factor	Category	Score if yes*
Congestive heart failure	Yes or no?	1
Hypertension	Yes or no?	1
Age (years)	<65	0
	65–74	1
	≥75	2
Diabetes mellitus	Yes or no?	1
History of stroke, transient ischemic attack or thromboembolic disease	Yes or no?	2
Vascular disease	Yes or no?	1
Female sex	Yes or no?	1

Table 7.11 The CHA_2DS_2-VASC score for estimating risk of stroke in patients with atrial fibrillation. *A total score of 0 indicates low annual stroke risk. Higher scores reflect increased risk. For example, total scores of 1, 2 and 3 equate to annual stroke risk of 1.3%, 2.2% and 3.2% respectively. A total score of 6 equates to a risk of 9.8%.

blocker or digoxin. A second agent can be added if control is suboptimal.

Digoxin is reserved for more sedentary patients because it can prevent increases in heart rate with exercise.

Clinical insight

Novel oral anticoagulants (NOACs) include factor Xa and thrombin inhibitors.

They are attractive because they appear to be as effective as warfarin in preventing venous thromboembolism in AF and do not require blood monitoring.

Management of acute atrial fibrillation

Emergency DCCV is required if there is significant cardiovascular compromise, regardless of AF duration. If AF occurs secondary to an acute systemic illness, the underlying cause is treated as a priority. If AF still persists, DCCV can be considered after ≥ 6 weeks of effective anticoagulation.

Management of paroxysmal atrial fibrillation

The frequency of paroxysms can be reduced by:

- Beta-blockers
- Class 1C drugs (flecanide or propafenone)
- Class 3 drugs (amiodarone or dronedarone).

However, these drugs are limited by contraindications, complications and lack of efficacy in some cases (see page 154).

DCCV DCCV can restore sinus rhythm, but reversion back to AF is common. Cardioversion carries a stroke risk and is avoided if AF lasts >48 h. DCCV is done only if ≥6 or more weeks of effective anticoagulation has been achieved, or if a transoesophageal echocardiogram excludes atrial thrombus.

Af ablation In paroxysmal AF, electrical isolation of the pulmonary veins via catheter ablation can be used to prevent recurrence. This can provide long-term relief but is invasive and often requires multiple attempts.

Pill-in-the-pocket This involves the patient taking a drug (usually a beta-blocker, flecanide or propafenone) if symptoms suggest recent onset of AF. It is an effective strategy in some patients.

Permanent atrial fibrillation

When sinus rhythm cannot be restored, the primary aim is to reduce the risk of thromboembolism. Rate control is indicated if the ventricular response is fast.

Prognosis

The prognosis for AF is good as long as the risk of thromboembolism is minimized and the rate is controlled.

Heart failure

Heart failure (HF) is a syndrome reflecting an inadequate circulation of blood due to impaired ventricular filling and/or ejection of blood. It has many causes and can be acute or chronic in nature. Coronary heart disease (CHD) is a common cause of both acute and chronic heart failure.

HF has a complex pathophysiology, often involving multiple compensatory mechanisms. The cardinal features of HF are dyspnea, fatigue and fluid retention. It also has many possible complications, including psychological, musculoskeletal, hematological, pulmonary, endocrine, endothelial, renal and hepatic dysfunction.

Echocardiography is used to assess both systolic and diastolic ventricular function and is the gold standard investigation for the diagnosis of HF. The underlying disease must be found and treated where possible.

8.1 Clinical scenario

Breathlessness at night, ankle swelling and cough

Presentation

Jeff Marks, aged 65 years, presents to his local emergency department with a 6-month history of nocturnal breathlessness and cough. He previously felt he merely had a series of colds, but made an appointment after his wife noticed that his ankles had begun to swell.

Diagnostic approach

Mr Marks has three common presenting complaints: shortness of breath, ankle swelling and cough (**Table 8.1**). Only heart, respiratory, renal or liver failure could cause all three simultaneously.

History

Mr Marks' illness started 6 months ago with what seemed like a heavy cold. This increased in intensity and he began experiencing a cough with white frothy sputum. He is not short

Symptom	Questions to ask	Associated symptoms	Possible differentials
Shortness of breath	Is it new? Is it getting worse? Is it just at night or during the day too? Does it come on with exertion, the cold, heavy meals? How many pillows does he use? Does the cough wake him?	Wheeze, chest pain and dizziness	HF, CHD, COPD and pulmonary embolus
Ankle swelling	When did this come on? Is it on one or both sides? Did it start after injury or surgery? Has it happened before? How far does it extend up the leg, and is it worsening?	Pain, redness and distended veins	Heart, renal or liver failure, lymphedema and deep venous thrombosis.
Cough	When does the cough occur? Is it productive? If so, what is the color and consistency of the sputum?	Green, frothy or blood stained	HF, infection, drug adverse effect, malignancy and anxiety

Table 8.1 Mr Marks' presenting features. CHD, coronary heart disease; COPD, chronic obstructive pulmonary disease.

Clinical insight

A patient's agenda must always be addressed, for example by considering:

- Ideas: what do they think is going on, and why?
- Concerns: what are their worries, and why?
- Expectations: what do they want?

of breath during the day, but wakes up breathless during the night and has difficulty lying flat.

He started to worry when his ankles began to swell. Mr Marks denies any palpitations, fever, weight loss or other symptoms.

His medical history includes:
- CHD – myocardial infarction treated with coronary artery bypass grafts (CABG) 5 years ago
- Hypertension
- Hypercholesterolemia
- Diabetes mellitus type 2.

He has had no angina since his CABG. He takes aspirin, atenolol, simvastatin, metformin and gliclazide. He is a retired bank clerk and has never smoked and currently does not drink alcohol. His systems review is unremarkable.

Diagnostic approach

Mr Marks has multiple risk factors for HF: CHD, diabetes and hypertension.

Chronic obstructive pulmonary disease (COPD) is unlikely as he has never smoked nor worked in a dusty environment. The absence of chest pain suggests that the symptoms are not ischemic in origin. The frothy white sputum strongly suggests pulmonary edema. Symptoms specific to the pulmonary edema of HF include:
- Paroxysmal nocturnal dyspnea – waking up breathless during the night
- Orthopnea – the inability to lie flat because of the resulting breathlessness.

Examination

- Mr Marks is apyrexial
- Heart rate – 110 beats/min
- Blood pressure – 100/80 mmHg
- Jugular venous pressure (JVP) is raised at 8 cm
- Capillary refill time is 2 seconds
- Respiratory rate is 20 breaths/min
- Oxygen saturation is 94% on room air.

A laterally displaced apex beat is found on precordial palpation. On auscultation, there are crepitations and reduced air entry at the bases and normal heart sounds. His ankles are swollen with fluid (edema) up to the mid shins.

Abdominal examination reveals moderate ascites and tender hepatomegaly.

Diagnostic approach

Mr Marks' tachycardia and hypotension indicate a reduced stroke volume due to impaired left ventricular function. Tachycardia is a compensatory attempt to meet peripheral circulatory demand. His normal capillary refill time suggests demand is being met.

His raised JVP reflects right ventricular impairment and elevated central venous pressure (CVP), possibly secondary to left ventricular failure. Right ventricular impairment leads to a build up of systemic fluid: ascites, ankle edema and liver swelling. Left ventricular impairment leads to pulmonary edema, evident as crepitations. Left ventricular failure leads to ventricular dilation, evident as a displaced apex beat.

The working diagnosis is congestive HF secondary to CHD.

Investigations

A chest X-ray shows cardiomegaly, pulmonary edema and pleural effusions (**Figure 8.1**).
An electrocardiogram (ECG) shows sinus tachycardia.

Baseline blood tests include full blood count; lipid profile; blood glucose; and tests of renal, thyroid and liver function and are all normal except for elevated transaminases, hyperbilirubinemia and hypoalbuminemia.

Diagnosis

Mr Marks is diagnosed with acute-on-chronic HF with reduced ejection fraction (HFREF) syndrome caused by left ventricular systolic dysfunction, most likely as a consequence of CHD. Ankle edema, a displaced apex beat and cardiomegaly are signs of chronic heart failure. His dilated, failing left ventricle has led to right-sided failure, as evident in the pulmonary edema seen on X-ray and his associated breathlessness. This is an acute exacerbation of long-standing disease.

Tachycardia occurs as the autonomic system attempts to compensate for insufficient cardiac output by an increase in heart rate.

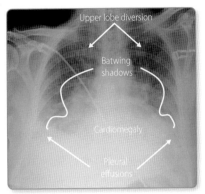

Figure 8.1 Chest X-ray showing the perihilar, batwing shadows of pulmonary edema. The increased cardiothoracic ratio (i.e. cardiac silhouette is >50% of the total width of the lungs) indicates cardiomegaly. Pleural effusions are a common sign of heart failure, but have many non-cardiac causes.

He is admitted to the coronary care unit for monitoring, intravenous diuretics and portable ECG to confirm the nature and severity of the left ventricular systolic dysfunction.

8.2 Chronic heart failure

Chronic HF is impaired ventricular filling and/or ejection with an onset over months to years.

It is classified by:

- Time – acute versus chronic
- Anatomy – right versus left
- Physiology – systolic versus diastolic
- Etiology – ischemic versus non-ischemic
- Genetics – inherited versus acquired
- Sequelae – low output versus high output.

Anatomy – right versus left

HF is categorized as to which side is affected. Congestive HF is when both sides are involved (i.e. biventricular HF). Rarely, isolated right ventricular failure occurs due to a massive pulmonary embolus or a inferior myocardial infarction.

Physiology – systolic versus diastolic

HF is also categorized by ejection fraction as this reflects different pathophysiologies and management:

- HF with reduced ejection fraction (HFREF) represents a failure of systolic ejection function (50% patients)
- HF with preserved ejection fraction (HFPEF) represents a failure of diastolic filling function (50% patients).

Functional classification NYHA functional classification is useful to gauge the impact on the patient's life and monitor disease progress or improvement (**Table 8.2**).

Clinical insight

Back pressure from left ventricular failure first affects the pulmonary system, causing pulmonary edema. This leads eventually to right ventricular failure and backpressure in the systemic circulation.

Disease progression stages The American College of Cardiology Foundation/American Heart Association (ACCF/AHA) 2013 guidelines provides criteria for staging HF disease progression (**Table 8.3**).

Epidemiology

HF affects about 1% of adults in Europe. Americans ≥40 years old have a 20% lifetime risk of developing HF. The average age of diagnosis is 76 years. HFREF is more common in men and HFPEF in women.

Diagnosis is assoicated with a 5-year survival rate of 50%, which is worse than that for many cancers. Heart failure is the most common cause of hospitalization in the over 65s, and is responsible for 5% of admissions.

Class	Symptoms	Limitations	Example
I	None	None	Normal activity
II	Mild	Slight	Breathless on incline
III	Moderate	Moderate	Comfortable only at rest
IV	Severe	Severe	Breathless even at rest

Table 8.2 New York Heart Association (NYHA) functional classification of heart failure.

Stage	Criteria	Example(s)
A	High risk without structural heart disease or symptoms	Type 2 diabetes mellitus Hypertension Obesity CHD Family medical history
B	Structural heart disease without signs or symptoms	Left ventricular hypertrophy Previous myocardial infarction Left ventricular systolic dysfunction
C	Structural heart disease with current or prior symptoms	Clinical HF
D	Refractory HF requiring specialist intervention	Transplant Organ support Palliation

Table 8.3 The American College of Cardiology Foundation/American Heart Association (ACCF/AHA) classification of the progression of HF.

Etiology

Any significant mechanical, structural or electrical cardiac abnormality can cause HF (**Table 8.4**). Non-cardiac causes, such as hematological, endocrine, inflammatory, infective or malignant disease, increase physiological demand on the heart.

Heart failure with reduced ejection fraction (HFREF) About 50% of HFREF is a consequence of CHD, typically myocardial infarction. *Non-ischemic* HFREF are mostly due to idiopathic dilated cardiomyopathy secondary to toxic, metabolic, infectious, valvular or arrhythmic causes.

Heart failure with preserved ejections fraction (HFPEF) HFPEF typically arises from a combination of hypertension, CHD, diabetes mellitus type 2 and obesity.

Cause of heart failure	Example of underlying cause	Ventricle affected	Incidence
Vascular dysfunction	CHD	Left	Common
Rhythm disturbance	Atrial fibrillation	Both	Common
Valvular dysfunction	Mitral regurgitation	Left	Common
Lifestyle	Obesity	Left	Common
Pulmonary disease	Pulmonary embolus	Right	Intermediate
Idiopathic	Dilated cardiomyopathy	Both	Intermediate
Infective	Viral myocarditis	Both	Rare
Infiltrative diseases	Amyloidosis	Both	Rare
Autoimmune disease	Hyperthyroidism	Both	Rare
Inherited	Atrial septal defect	Right	Rare
Drug adverse effect	Bleomycin chemotherapy	Both	Rare
Physiological state	Post-partum cardiomyopathy	Both	Rare

Table 8.4 Causes of heart failure.

> **Clinical insight**
>
> Encourage all cardiac patients to improve their lifestyle. Cardiovascular risk is reduced by stopping smoking, taking regular exercise and losing weight.

Prevention

Primary prevention includes early recognition of and interventions to reduce cardiovascular risk factors, e.g. hypertension, diabetes mellitus type 2, obesity and hypercholesterolemia. The aim is to reduce the risk of myocardial infarction, which leads to HFREF, and left ventricular hypertrophy (LVH), which leads to HFPEF.

Secondary prevention focuses on early recognition and intervention to reduce ischemic injury and prevent adverse myocardial remodeling.

Pathogenesis

HFREF and HFPEF have different pathogenic mechanisms leading to distinct pathophysiologies (**Figure 8.2**).

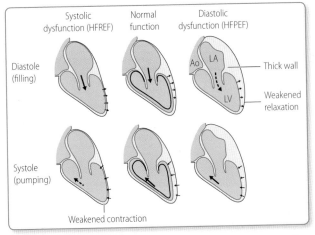

Figure 8.2 The pathophysiology of heart failure in the left atrium and ventricle. Heart failure with reduced ejection fraction (HFREF) represents systolic dysfunction: reduced contraction of the heart during systole. Heart failure with preserved ejection fraction (HFPEF) represents diastolic dysfunction with reduced relaxation of the heart during diastole. Both lead to reduced stroke volume. Ao, aorta; LA, left atrium; LV, left ventricle.

HFREF This is caused by an abnormality of systolic contraction, i.e. left ventricular systolic dysfunction. For example, myocardial infarction leads to cell death, tissue necrosis and scar formation. Scar tissue reduces stroke volume, and disrupts the optimal length–tension relationship of the myocardium, according to the Frank–Starling law (**Figure 8.3;** see also page 45).

In a healthy heart:
- Increasing venous return increases preload
- Increased myocardial stretch increases the number of actin–myosin interactions
- Increased end-diastolic volume
- Increased stroke volume.

In the failing heart, after a certain point, the increased stretch only over-stretches the myocardium beyond its optimum length–tension relationship, reducing its contractile force.

Figure 8.3 The Frank–Starling law. ① healthy individual during exercise and ② at rest; ③ heart failure; ④ cardiogenic shock. Heart contractility (stroke volume) normally responds to increases in venous return (i.e. end-diastolic volume). This does not occur adequately in patients with heart failure.

HFPEF This is caused by an abnormality of myocardial relaxation, i.e. left ventricular diastolic dysfunction. Hypertension, for example, increases left ventricular afterload and chronically leads to compensatory LVH. This creates a thick ventricular wall and a small ventricular cavity. The increased stiffness and reduced compliance mean that the left ventricle fails to relax during diastole.

Myocardial fibrosis may also occur, due to subclinical microvascular ischemia, causing:

- Increased left ventricular end-diastolic pressure
- Inadequate filling of the ventricle
- Reduced stroke volume (and therefore cardiac output).

Compensation Both HFREF and HFPEF reduce cardiac output (**Figure 8.2**). This leads to up-regulation of the sympathetic nervous system and the renin–angiotensin–aldosterone system (RAAS), increasing cardiac output, total peripheral resistance, and blood pressure. This initially augments the failing heart to maintain perfusion, but once cardiac function deteriorates beyond a point, they hasten its decline (**Figure 8.4**).

Clinical features

Patients present with (**Figure 8.5, Table 8.5**):

- Fluid retention, e.g. pulmonary and ankle edema
- Signs of compensation, e.g. tachycardia
- Cachexia due to a catabolic state, reduced tissue perfusion and inflammation.

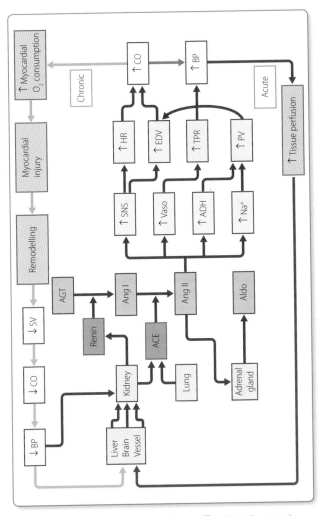

Figure 8.4 The pathophysiology of heart failure. ACE, angiotensin-converting enzyme; ADH, antidiuretic hormone; AGT, angiotensinogen; Aldo, aldosterone; Ang I, angiotensin I; Ang II, angiotensin II; BP, blood pressure; CO, cardiac output; EDV, end-diastolic volume; HR, heart rate; PV, plasma volume; SNS, sympathetic nervous system; SV, stroke volume; TPR, total peripheral resistance; Vaso, vasoconstriction.

Figure 8.5 Common signs of heart failure.

Clinical features	Sensitivity (%)	Specificity (%)
Symptom:		
Orthopnea	21	81
Edema	23	80
Paroxysmal nocturnal dyspnea	33	76
Dyspnea	66	52
Signs:		
Tachycardia	7	99
Raised jugular venous pressure	10	97
Third heart sound	31	95
Periheral edema	10	93

Table 8.5 Clinical features of heart failure and their sensitivity and specificity.

Right-sided HF is associated with features of raised systemic venous pressure (e.g. peripheral edema and elevated JVP) and left-sided HF is associated with increased left atrial and pulmonary pressure (e.g. pulmonary

> ## Clinical insight
>
> **Non-cardiogenic pulmonary edema** is caused by, high altitude, decreased plasma oncotic pressure as a result of low albumin and increased alveolar capillary permeability in acute respiratory distress syndrome

edema and resultant dyspnea) (**Table 8.6**). The degree of breathlessness is a key aspect of the NYHA functional classification (**Table 8.2**).

Investigations

All patients require blood tests, ECG, chest X-ray and echocardiography. Exercise tests are also commonly performed to inform management and prognosis.

Coronary angiography may also be done to assess for CHD, the commonest cause of HFREF.

Blood tests Blood tests are performed to rule out other causes of breathlessness, e.g. anemia, and assess severity; e.g. brain natriuretic peptide (BNP) is a marker of disease severity (**Table 8.7**).

Symptom or sign	Right-sided heart failure	Left-sided heart failure
Peripheral edema	Prominent	Not prominent
Edema	Systemic	Pulmonary
Organomegaly	Liver	Cardiac
Raised jugular venous pressure	Prominent	Not prominent
Dyspnea	Not prominent	Prominent
Gastrointestinal	Prominent	Not prominent

Table 8.6 Clinical features of right-sided and left-sided heart failure.

Electrocardiography Common abnormalities seen on ECG include:
- CHD: Q waves, T wave inversion, prolonged QRS [i.e. bundle branch block (BBB)]
- LVH, especially in HFPEF
- Prolonged QRS duration (i.e. BBB) – a marker of severity
- Arrhythmias: atrial fibrillation, paroxysmal ventricular arrhythmias.

Chest X-ray Chest X-ray may show (**Figures 8.1 and 8.6**):
- Pleural effusions of fluid accumulating between the layers of pleura
- Kerley B lines from fluid accumulating between the interlobular septa
- Bilateral perihilar markings (classically batwing-shaped) from the collection of alveolar fluid
- Upper zone venous vessel enlargement from pulmonary venous hypertension
- Cardiomegaly: increased cardiothoracic ratio (> 50%).

Echocardiography Echocardiography is performed on diagnosis to:
- Measure the ejection fraction and distinguish HFREF and HFPEF
- Assess valves

Blood test	Assessing for
Full blood count	Anemia or infection
Urea and electrolytes	Renal failure
Liver function tests	Liver failure
Thyroid function tests	Thyroid disease
Lipid profile	Hypercholesterolemia
Glucose	Diabetes mellitus
Natriuretic peptides	Disease severity

Table 8.7 Blood tests in patients with suspected heart failure.

Figure 8.6 Chest X-ray features of heart failure: (1) Kerley B lines (2) upper lobe venous diversion (3) ill-defined peri-hilar (batswings) shadowing (4) fluid in the oblique and horizontal fissures (5) pleural effusions (6) increased cardiothoracic ratio, where the width of the heart shadow (H) is >50% of the width of the lung fields (L).

- Measure chambers
- Identify LVH.

An echocardiogram showing normal systolic function does not exclude HF. There may still be:

- Valve disease
- Diastolic dysfunction
- Pericardial disease
- High-output HF.

> ### Clinical insight
>
> Patients can be shocked by a diagnosis of heart failure, particularly by the term 'failure'. Conversely, if their symptoms are mild, some may not comprehend the seriousness of the diagnosis

Magnetic resonance imaging Cardiac magnetic resonance imaging (MRI) can provide high-resolution structural and functional assessment of:

- Ventricular volumes
- Wall thickness
- Chamber dimensions
- Ventricular systolic functions
- Myocardial ischemia
- Myocardial scarring
- Infiltrative disease.

Exercise tests These include the 6-minute walk test to assess functional capacity and monitor progress, and cardiopulmonary exercise testing to assess exercise capacity, inform prognosis and assess the need for heart transplant.

Clinical insight

An increased concentration of brain natriuretic protein (> 400 pg/mL) strongly suggests heart failure. BNP is released by myocardium in response to stretch. It increases renal natriuresis and causes vasodilation, thereby decreasing blood pressure.

Management

Lifestyle modification, medication and device therapy aim to:

- Treat the cause
- Reduce symptoms
- Reduce aggravating factors
- Improve prognosis and quality of life.

Key evidence-based therapy recommendations of the 2013 ACCF/AHA guidelines are shown in **Table 8.8**.

Lifestyle modification

All patients should be encouraged to (see pages 146 and 306):

- Exercise – a tailored rehabilitation program of structured aerobic exercise is safe in stable patients, improves functional capacity, quality of life and reduces morbidity
- Moderate alcohol intake; abstain in alcohol cardiomyopathy

Stage	Recommended therapy
A	Control HTN and dyslipidemia in accordance with HTN guidelines to lower HF risk
	Control other risk factors: obesity, diabetes, smoking
B	ACEI (ARB if ACEI not tolerated) + beta-blocker for patients with • Reduced EF + previous ACS or MI (↓ HF symptoms, ↓ mortality) • Reduced EF without previous MI (↓ HF symptoms)
	Statins for patients with • ACS history (↓ HF symptoms, ↓ CV events)
	BP control in accordance with HTN guidelines for patients with • Structural heart changes and no ACS history (↓ HF symptoms)

Table 8.8 *Continued*

C		Specific patient education to self-manage HF care
		Exercise training is safe to improve functional status
		Long-term anticoagulant therapy in patients with AF and another cardioembolic risk factor (HTN, diabetes, CVA history, ≥75 years). Choice of agent depends on patient's clinical profile
	HFREF	Pharmacological measures as listed for A and B (↓ morbidity, ↓ mortality), i.e. ACEI (or ARB) + beta-blocker *plus, if needed*: • Loop diuretic if volume overloaded in NYHA class II–IV • Hydralazine + nitrate if still symptomatic African American and NYHA class III–IV • Aldosterone antagonist if no CKD and patient is in NYHA class II–IV with LVEF ≤35% (↓ morbidity, ↓ mortality) or is post MI with LVEF ≤40% and HF symptoms or diabetes
		ICD therapy (↓ mortality from sudden cardiac death) in patients with HREF at >40 days after MI *and*: • Non-ischemic dilated cardiomyopathy or CHD, with both LVEF ≤35% and NYHA class II or III symptoms • LVEF ≤30% and NYHA class I
		Cardiac resynchronization therapy for patients with LVEF ≤35%, LBBB with QRS ≥150 ms and NYHA class II, III or ambulatory IV symptoms
	HFPEF	Systolic and diastolic BP control
		Diuretics to relieve volume overload symptoms
D		Treat cardiogenic shock with IV inotropic support until definitive treatment
		Cardiac transplantation

Table 8.8 Key treatment recommendations for heart failure stages A to D: treatments with class I evidence in the 2013 ACCF/AHA heart failure guidelines. ACEI, angiotensin-converting enzyme inhibitor; ACS, acute coronary syndrome; AF, atrial fibrillation; ARB, angiotensin II receptor blocker; CHD, coronary heart disease; CKD, chronic kidney disease; CVA, cerebrovascular accident; EF, ejection fraction; HTN, hypertension; ICD, Implantable cardioverter-defibrillator ; LVEF, left ventricular EF; NYHA, New York Heart Association; MI, myocardial infarction.

- Quit smoking
- Restrict fluid (to < 1.5 L/day) and salt (to <6 g/day) intake to minimize fluid retention symptoms. Advise patients to monitor their weight and seek medical advice if it increases > 2 kg in 2 days
- Receive vaccinations: influenza (yearly) and pneumococcus (once).

Patients should be made aware of driving restrictions.

> ## Clinical insight
>
> Heart failure is a syndrome not a diagnosis. The underlying cause must be investigated and treated.

Medication

Medications can improve symptoms, prognosis and target underlying cause.

HFREF First-line treatment for all patients is a beta-blocker and an angiotensin-converting enzyme (ACE) inhibitor. Patients are started on low doses and titrated until stable. Long-term monitoring is performed in primary care.

A diuretic is prescribed in proportion to symptoms to relieve fluid retention and congestion. Patients should be monitored for renal function and electrolyte derangement when dosages are started or changed.

Digoxin is used to control heart rate in patients with atrial fibrillation or advanced HF.

Aldosterone antagonists, such as spironolactone, reduce mortality and morbidity by reducing myocardial fibrosis and improving vascular function.

HFPEF No medications target HFPEF pathophysiology or are proven to improve prognosis. Treatment therefore involves aggressive management of underlying hypertension, diabetes, weight control and lipid control.

Diuretics reduce symptoms of fluid retention and beta-blockers reduce heart rate and increase diastole.

Devices

Cardiac resynchronization therapy and implantable cardioverter defibrillators improve prognosis for HFREF patients whose heart chambers contract dyssynchronously or who are prone to life-threatening ventricular arrhythmias (see page 274).

Surgical management

Primary valve disease indicates valve repair or replacement, and CABG is indicated in those with severe CHD.

Clinical insight

Depression is common in patients with heart failure and generally correlates with disease severity. Physicians need to directly ascertain if patients are depressed, as outcomes are worse in patients with untreated depression.

Patients with severe symptoms despite medical therapy (i.e. NYHA class 3 or 4) may be considered for:
- Mitral valve repair for mitral regurgitation
- Left ventricular restoration
- Insertion of a left ventricular assist device (**Figure 8.7**)
- Heart transplant – the only curative option.

Heart transplant is contraindicated in the elderly, renal failure, irreversible pulmonary arterial hypertension and other severe non-cardiac disease.

Prognosis

The prognosis for chronic HF is worse than the prognosis for many cancers. Around 35% of patients with a new diagnosis will die within 12 months, and approximately 50% in 5 years.

Figure 8.7 A left ventricular assist device in situ.

Aorta

Pulmonary arteries

Left atrium

Left ventricle

Left ventricular assist device

Severely symptomatic (NYHA class 4 or ACCF/AHA stage D) patients with a poor prognosis, likely require palliative care.

8.3 Acute heart failure

Chronic HF symptoms appear slowly over time and worsen gradually. In acute HF, symptoms develop suddenly and are initially severe.

65% have acute-on-chronic HF, 30% have new (*de novo*) disease, and 5% are nearing the end of their life.

Epidemiology

Patients are typically in their mid-seventies. Half of cases have HFREF, and half have HFPEF. Two thirds of patients are known to have CHD, and one third have diabetes, chronic kidney disease, COPD or atrial fibrillation.

Etiology

Common causes of *de novo* failure include myocardial infarction, acute valvular dysfunction, arrhythmia, cardiac tamponade, medications (e.g. NSAIDs), IV fluids or thyroid dysfunction.

Acute-on-chronic HF occurs with decompensation, for example, due to severe illness (e.g. infection or anemia), negatively inotropic drugs, non-concordance with medication or thyroid dysfunction.

Prevention

Prevention measures include:
- Adequate monitoring
- Ensuring medication concordance
- Detecting and treating arrhythmia early
- Managing intercurrent illnesses (e.g. pneumonia) or comorbidities aggressively.

Clinical features

Patients present with fatigue, edema, cough, breathlessness and severe orthopnea.

Signs include tachycardia, tachypnea, hypertension (**Table 8.9**) and a third heart sound. Signs of fluid status and tissue perfusion are used to guide treatment (**Table 8.10**). An elevated JVP and peripheral edema are commonly seen and reflect right-sided decompensation.

Severe presentations are usually a result of left-sided failure causing severe pulmonary edema, evident as reduced oxygen saturations and inspiratory crepitations.

Investigations
All acutely ill patients are assessed using resuscitation guidelines (e.g. the ABCDE approach) to prioritize treatment.

Investigations are the same as for suspected chronic HF, but with an emphasis on urgent echocardiography (where available) if the diagnosis is unknown.

ECG changes are usually non-specific, but chest X-ray will demonstrate pulmonary edema (**Figure 8.1**).

Management
Management is determined by hemodynamic state and clinical stage (**Table 8.10**). Once stable, therapy for chronic HF is started.

Medication Initial management, ideally in a coronary

> ## Clinical insight
>
> In cardiogenic shock the heart is unable to pump enough blood for the body's basic needs. It is defined as SBP < 90 mmHg in the presence of low urine output, poor peripheral perfusion, confusion or lactate > 2.0 mmol/L.

Blood pressure	Prevalence (% of cases)	Presentation
High (> 150 mmHg)	50	Symptoms with abrupt onset (hours or days)
Normal (120–149 mmHg)	40	Symptoms with gradual onset (days or weeks)
Low (91–119 mmHg)	9	Hypoperfusion
Very low (< 90 mmHg)	1	Cardiogenic shock

Table 8.9 Blood pressure in patients with acute severe *de novo* heart failure.

Hemodynamic state	Treatment
Wet and cold	Vasodilators and additional diuretics
Wet and warm	Diuretics and additional vasodilators
Cold and dry	Ionotropes and intra-aortic balloon pump
Warm and dry	The aim for all patients with heart failure

Table 8.10 Treatment of patients with acute heart failure in various hemodynamic and clinical states. Wet, signs of fluid overload; dry, absence of these; cold, signs of reduced tissue perfusion; warm, absence of these.

Clinical insight

Breathless patients with normal oxygen saturation (94–98%) are not given oxygen as there is no evidence of benefit.

care unit or high-dependency unit, includes:
- IV loop diuretic to remove excess fluid
- IV morphine to reduce stress and to venodilate
- IV glyceryl trinitrate to vasodilate and accommodate excess fluid
- Cessation of administration of inappropriate drugs (e.g. NSAIDs)
- Inotropes to augment cardiac output where a reversible cause of cardiogenic shock is identified.

Non-pharmacological management Initial management also includes:
- Sitting patient up
- Stop IV fluids (except in acute right ventricular failure)
- Oxygen if hypoxic (saturations < 94%)
- Continuous positive airway pressure (CPAP) ventilation in patients with pulmonary edema and significant dyspnea and hypoxia
- Monitoring of fluid balance: urea, electrolytes, urine output and body weight
- Fluid intake restricted to <1.5 L/day
- Invasive ventilation if respiratory failure occurs.

Prevention of cardiovascular disease

Despite decreasing mortality attributable to cardiovascular disease (CVD) in the developed world, the global incidence is increasing. This is due to both increasing incidence in the developing world and ageing populations. Coronary heart disease (CHD) is the most preventable form of CVD, and is predicted to be the primary cause of global morbidity and mortality by 2020.

Primary prevention is intervention before atherosclerotic disease is clinically evident. This focuses on diet, lifestyle education, management plans and medical interventions to lower cardiovascular risk factors. Atherosclerosis can be slowed and even reversed by changes in diet and lifestyle. However, recent evidence suggests health promotion via counseling and education produces only mild reductions in risk factors, with marginal impact on CHD morbidity and mortality. The main benefit is seen in high-risk hypertensive and diabetic patients.

Secondary prevention is aimed at the early detection and treatment of all atherosclerotic disease. Peripheral vascular disease is under-recognized as a forerunner and comorbidity of CHD.

9.1 Preventive measures

Calculating cardiovascular risk

Primary prevention hinges on an assessment of cardiovascular risk. Risk factors are categorized as non-modifiable, modifiable and emerging (lipid and inflammatory markers) (**Table 9.1**). Most are atherogenic, i.e. they increase the amount or rate of atherosclerosis in arteries. The 3 major modifiable factors are smoking, hyperlipidemia and hypertension.

Risk score calculators (e.g. www.qrisk.org) use data from large population studies to predict the risk of a future cardiovascular event (see page 145). Most report a person's 10-year risk; 20% or over is usually considered high risk and indicates primary prevention strategies should be adopted.

Class	Risk factors
Modifiable	Smoking, physical inactivity, atherogenic diet, BMI ≥25, hypertension (e.g. BP >140/90 mmHg), hyperlipidemia (e.g. total cholesterol <5 mmol/L/190 mg/dL), stress
Non-modifiable	Age, sex, family history/genetic
Emerging	C-reactive protein, fibrinogen, homocysteine, arterial calcification, lipoprotein(a)

Table 9.1 Cardiovascular risk factors. BMI, body mass index. BP, blood pressure.

Clinical insight

C-reactive protein (CRP) is an acute phase protein produced by the liver, and correlates with levels of systemic inflammation. Atherosclerosis is a systemic inflammatory and metabolic disease.

Risk calculations are used to guide treatment intensity and monitor progress. As many interventions are behavioral, it is essential to promote patient understanding and involvement in setting and making risk calculation targets.

Patients who are already high-risk, and therefore unsuitable for many risk calculators, include those over 75 or with proven:

- Atherosclerosis
- Hypertension
- Diabetes mellitus type 1 or 2
- Renal dysfunction
- Inherited dyslipidemia.

Risk factor reduction

Interventions aim to reduce modifiable risk factors:

- Smoking cessation
- Physical activity – at least 30 minutes, five times a week
- Healthy eating
- Maintain a healthy body weight [body-mass index (BMI) <25 kg/m^2]
- BP <140/90 mmHg
- Total cholesterol <5 mmol/L (190 mg/dL)
- Normal glucose metabolism

- Avoidance of stress
- Antiplatelet medication (e.g. aspirin).

Primary interventions should begin with diet and weight decrease, an increase in physical activity and smoking cessation.

Behavioral change

There are three levels to encouraging behavioral change in patients:

- Brief advice: opportunistic conversation raising patient awareness and assessing their desire to change
- Brief interventions: structured advice providing more formal help, e.g. arranging targets and follow up
- Motivational interviewing to examine their motivation and help them take action. This involves listening and patient-centered counseling skills that support patients to explore their ambivalence about changing their health-related behaviors (**Figure 9.1**).

Smoking

Smoking is decreasing in much of the developed world, but still increasing in the developing world. It is the leading preventable cause of CVD.

Smoking is atherogenic as it causes endothelial cell dysfunction, an increase in platelet and macrophage adherence to the endothelium, is prothrombotic and proinflammatory, and it induces tissue remodeling.

Smoking cessation is proven to be beneficial in established atherosclerosis as stopping smoking can lead to a reduction in atherosclerotic burden. It is also effective in secondary prevention, with significant reduction in 5-year mortality post MI or in patients with known CHD.

Physical activity

A sedentary lifestyle is associated with urbanization and a western lifestyle. It increases coagulopathy, decreases cardiovascular fitness and is associated with depression, obesity, type 2 diabetes and metabolic syndrome.

A common goal is 30–60 minutes of exercise of sufficient intensity to cause shortness of breath, 3–5 times a week

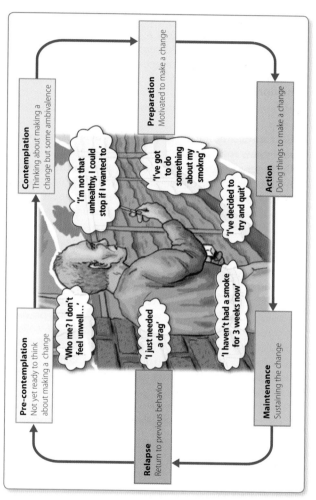

Figure 9.1 Motivational interviewing as informed by Prochaska and DiClemente's model of behavioral change. This example concerns smoking cessation but the theory is applicable to any behavior.

(see page 146). Secondary prevention often requires detailed programs and medical supervision for high-risk patients.

Diet

An unhealthy diet is atherogenic due to high fat and salt intake and is associated with being overweight or obese, and with type 2 diabetes and metabolic syndrome. A healthy diet is therefore the cornerstone of CVD prevention.

Specific diet education and plans may be needed (**Table 9.2**), though exact recommendations vary. A healthy cardiovascular diet includes daily whole grains, nuts, unsaturated fats, fruit and vegetables, fish and moderate (1–2 units) alcohol intake (see page 147).

Component	ESC recommendation	AHA/ACC recommendation
Saturated fatty acids	< 10% calories	5–6% calories
Trans unsaturated fatty acids	As little as possible	Reduce
Salt	<5 g/day	Reduce (e.g. <2.4 g/day if hypertensive)
Fiber	30–45 g/day	Diet emphasizes intake of vegetables, fruits, and whole grains; includes low-fat dairy products, poultry, fish, legumes, nontropical vegetable oils, and nuts; with limited intake of sweets, sugar-sweetened beverages, and red meat
Fruit	200 g/day (2–3 servings)	
Vegetables	200 g/day (2–3 servings)	
Fish	Twice a week (≥1 oily)	
Alcohol	♀≤ 1 glass (20 g)/day ♂≤ 2 glasses (20 g)/day	Average of: ♀ ≤1 glass (20 g)/day ♂ ≤2 glasses (20 g)/day

Table 9.2 Guidelines for diet proportions to prevent cardiovascular disease. Based on the European Society of Cardiology (ESC) 2012 guidelines and the American Heart Association/American College of Cardiology (AHA/ACC) 2014 guidelines.

> **Clinical insight**
>
> Garlic slightly lowers cholesterol, inhibits platelet aggregation and may lower blood pressure

Weight

Obesity is approaching global epidemic proportions. It is associated with CVD, hypertension, type 2 diabetes, metabolic syndrome, dyslipidemia, raised inflammatory markers, certain cancers, Alzheimer's disease and sleep apnea.

Although commonly measured in BMI, central obesity, i.e. an increased waist-to-hip circumference or waist-to-weight ratio, is a stronger risk factor for CHD (**Table 9.3**).

Blood pressure

Hypertension is the most common risk factor for CVD and should be screened for whenever possible. The increased stress on arterial walls increases arterial damage, inflammation and atherogenesis. A reduction in diastolic blood pressure by 6 mmHg leads to a 15% decrease in CHD risk, and a 42% decrease in cerebrovascular accident risk. Isolated systolic hypertension is also a major risk factor for IHD.

Recommended targets are <140/90 mmHg or <130/80 mmHg in chronic kidney disease.

Weight	BMI (kg/m²)	CHD risk	
		Waist circumference ≤102 cm/≤88 cm	Waist circumference >102 cm/>88 cm
Underweight	<18.5	…	…
Normal	18.5–24.9	…	…
Overweight	25.0–29.9	↑	↑ ↑
Obesity, class I	30.0–34.9	↑ ↑	↑ ↑ ↑
II	35.0–39.9	↑ ↑ ↑	↑ ↑ ↑
III	≥40	↑ ↑ ↑ ↑	↑ ↑ ↑ ↑

Table 9.3 The increased risk of coronary heart disease (CHD) in overweight and obese people. BMI, body mass index.

Self-monitoring and management of hypertension is important in primary and secondary prevention of CHD. Central to this is clear communication with patients and support from medical professionals.

> ## Clinical insight
>
> The metabolic syndrome includes any three of:
> - Abdominal obesity
> - Low HDL
> - Hypertension
> - Fasting hyperglycemia
> - Hypertriglyceridemia
>
> Its prevalence in the US is >20% of persons ≥20 years old and >40% of those >40 years.

Therapy targets The patient's cardiovascular risk score, blood pressure and evidence of end organ damage guide management (**Figure 4.2**).

Salt reduction initiatives Population-wide programs to reduce salt intake are considered one of the simplest and most cost-effective ways to reduce blood pressure and improve global public health. They involve food industry regulations and package labeling. Most countries with salt reduction programs have maximum intake targets of 5–8 g/day. The average intake in the UK, for example, in 2011 was 8.1 g/day. It is estimated by the Consensus Action on Salt and Health (CASH) in the UK, that a reduction to 6 g/day would decrease the average risk of myocardial infarction by 16% and cerebrovascular accident risk by 22%.

Lipids

High levels of low-density lipoprotein (LDL) cholesterol are atherogenic (see page 173). Elevated triglycerides also increase risk.

Screening or investigation of CHD involves a full fasting lipid profile. A key risk indicator appears to be the ratio of total or LDL cholesterol to high-density lipoprotein (HDL).

Familial hypercholesterolemia Familial hypercholesterolamia should be excluded if the patient has a strong family history of premature CHD (see page 217). It is an autosomal dominant inherited disorder of cholesterol metabolism. It is undiagnosed in as many as 90% of patients because cholesterol is often not checked in people under 40 years old.

Early identification with a simple fasting lipid blood test is important to allow prompt treatment. All patients with definite, possible or suspected familial hyperlipidemia are referred to a specialist center for diagnosis and management.

Therapy targets Therapy aims to decrease LDL cholesterol and increase HDL cholesterol. This is achieved by medication (statins in the first instance), a healthy diet and increase in physical activity. Most recent guidelines do not recommend specific treatment targets for primary prevention, but recommend assessing the individual patient's clinical findings, lipid profile and family history. The European Society of Cardiology 2011 targets are given in **Table 5.5**.

The UK's National Institute for Health and Care Excellence (NICE) recommends a target LDL of <2.0 mmol/L (<~100 mg/dL) in secondary prevention.

Statins Statins exert their effects in the liver and are very effective at lowering LDL cholesterol.

They are uniformly prescribed to patients with CHD, regardless of starting cholesterol level, because they reduce cardiac events and total mortality. If a single agent does not control lipid levels, combination therapy is required.

> ## Clinical insight
>
> Statin side effects include myositis (i.e. muscle aches), rhabdomyolysis, cataracts, kidney failure, and moderate or severe liver dysfunction.

Diabetes

Uncontrolled diabetes is a pro-inflammatory and pro-infective state. A person with diabetes has a two-fold greater absolute risk of CVD than a non-diabetic.

It is atherogenic due to glucose disruption of structural proteins, largely via the formation of advanced glycation end-products: permanent bonding to and disruption of proteins (e.g. hemoglobin A1c (HbA1c)). This includes structural proteins of small vessels (i.e. microvascular disease) and the walls of larger arteries, which promotes atherosclerosis – macrovascular diabetic disease.

CHD prevention in diabetic patients requires aggressive management of diabetes and of all cardiovascular risk factors: weight management, physical activity, blood pressure and cholesterol. Targets are often lower than for non-diabetics.

Stress

Although there is mixed evidence on the link between stress and CHD, there is a strong association with depression, social isolation and poor social support.

Chronic neurohormonal activation increases heart rate and blood pressure: life events, work stress, anxiety, type A personality traits. Consistently raised cortisol inhibits immune housekeeping function, which can promote arterial wall damage. In western cultures, stress is also associated with poor diet, low socioeconomic status, smoking, increased alcohol intake and lack of physical activity.

Acute stress and anxiety can promote arrhythmias, a pro-thrombotic state and an CHD event in established disease.

Aspirin

Aspirin decreases the risk of a first MI by a quarter to a third. Primary prevention in those with a 10% 10 year risk involves low dose (e.g. 75 mg) aspirin. It is also beneficial in secondary prevention of MI and ischemic stroke.

The increased risk of gastrointestinal or cerebrovascular bleeding must be considered.

9.2 Secondary prevention/cardiac rehabilitation

Secondary intervention includes regular blood pressure checks, monitoring of fasting lipids, and diet and lifestyle advice, as well as medications including aspirin, statins, ACE inhibitors, and beta-blockers.

Cardiac rehabilitation provides continued information and support to achieve the many lifestyle modifications required after a heart attack. Patients are able to meet in groups over a period of several weeks and are given a supervised exercise program. This allows them to meet other people who have been through the same experience and to regain confidence in getting back to a full and active lifestyle. Use of expert patient or patient forum services can also be a valuable source of information and support.

Management of stable angina

Stable angina represents stable CHD (see page 225). All patients with new-onset chest pain with a possible ischemic cause are referred for further investigation. In the interim, patients should be immediately started on aspirin 75 mg once daily, and should undergo the following investigations:

- ECG to look for evidence of ischemia
- Fasting lipid profile
- Hemoglobin A1c.

Secondary prevention is started as soon as possible. Many patients require a lipid-lowering agent, preferably a statin (these drugs are thought to have pleiotropic effects). If a patient has angina attacks more than twice a week, regular anti-anginal medication is started and the patient is referred to a cardiologist for further assessment.

Index

Note: Page numbers in **bold** or *italic* refer to tables or figures respectively.